Praise for Clinical Research Manual

"If the changing landscape of clinical research has bewildered you, Cavalieri and Rupp's book is the key to enlightenment. Their sensible and matter-of-fact guidance prepares investigators and research personnel to launch careers in clinical research or to pursue innovative strategies to enhance the performance of research sites. A wealth of templates, tools, and practical tips makes the *Clinical Research Manual* a valuable reference for research professionals. After 25 years of experience in clinical research administration, I am inspired by the authors' commitment to foster the future of clinical research through sharing their knowledge and expertise."

–Carol Fedor, RN, ND, CCRC
Director, Human Research Protection Program
Center for Clinical Research
University Hospitals Case Medical Center

"This book is long overdue! Cavalieri and Rupp have combined their knowledge and broad research experience to write a manual that is useful for all members of the clinical research team. *Clinical Research Manual: Practical Tools and Templates for Managing Clinical Research* provides a framework for a consistent approach to all aspects of conducting clinical trials. Up to now, many research team members learned these things by trial and error. This book is a must have for every clinical research team."

–Joan M. Lappe, PhD, RN, FAAN
Criss/Beirne Professor of Nursing
Professor of Medicine
Creighton University

"An invaluable resource for clinical research professionals, whether they are new to the discipline or have a long history of clinical trial experience. The format of the manual allows the reader to 'hopscotch' to topics of interest, gaining insights from the authors via practical tips and templates. Cavalieri and Rupp effectively take the point of view of the researcher, anticipating the challenges researchers are likely to encounter in the preparation and conduct of clinical trials."

–Art Gertel, MS
VP, Strategic Regulatory Consulting & Medical Affairs
TFS Americas

"Cavalieri and Rupp clearly possess a wealth of practical knowledge regarding the conduct of clinical trials and demonstrate their decades of experience through their practical examples and tips. The information conveyed is readily translatable to practice and is presented in a straightforward and easy-to-use format for those who work in the clinical research field."

–*Christopher J. Kratochvil, MD*
Associate Vice Chancellor for Clinical Research,
University of Nebraska Medical Center
Chief Medical Officer, UNeHealth

"The *Clinical Research Manual* should be lauded as truly the how-to manual on the intricacies of clinical trials research for individuals across a variety of specialties. The authors' 20 years of experience in clinical trials research is brought forward in a simple, straightforward manner that captures the detailed activity across this research continuum. It offers practical advice and guidance for the more experienced as well as the novice learner. This manual highlights the need for collaborative, engaging methodologies of the various stakeholders whose participation and expertise become the linchpin of any trial's success. It is incredibly comprehensive, leaving no stone unturned and emphasizing points with applicable examples. Anyone entering this arena would benefit greatly from this manual, as well as individuals who just need to understand an element of clinical trials research a bit more specifically. My congratulations to the authors for creating a manual that is easy to use, yet powerful in its content and references."

–*Rosanna D. Morris, BSN, RN, MBA, NE-BC*
Senior Vice President Patient Care Services, Chief Nursing Officer
The Nebraska Medical Center

Clinical Research Manual

Practical Tools and Templates for Managing Clinical Research

R. Jennifer Cavalieri, BSN, RN, CCRC, CCRP

Mark E. Rupp, MD

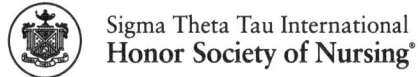
Sigma Theta Tau International
Honor Society of Nursing

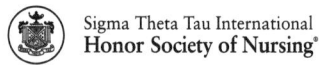
Sigma Theta Tau International
Honor Society of Nursing®

Copyright © 2013 by Sigma Theta Tau International

All rights reserved. This book is protected by copyright. No part of it may be reproduced, stored in a retrieval system, or transmitted in any form or by any means, electronic, mechanical, photocopying, recording, or otherwise, without written permission from the publisher. Any trademarks, service marks, design rights, or similar rights that are mentioned, used, or cited in this book are the property of their respective owners. Their use here does not imply that you may use them for similar or any other purpose.

The Honor Society of Nursing, Sigma Theta Tau International (STTI) is a nonprofit organization whose mission is to support the learning, knowledge, and professional development of nurses committed to making a difference in health worldwide. Founded in 1922, STTI has more than 130,000 active members in more than 85 countries. Members include practicing nurses, instructors, researchers, policymakers, entrepreneurs, and others. STTI's 488 chapters are located at 668 institutions of higher education throughout Australia, Botswana, Brazil, Canada, Colombia, England, Ghana, Hong Kong, Japan, Kenya, Malawi, Mexico, the Netherlands, Pakistan, Singapore, South Africa, South Korea, Swaziland, Sweden, Taiwan, Tanzania, the United States, and Wales. More information about STTI can be found online at www.nursingsociety.org.

Sigma Theta Tau International
550 West North Street
Indianapolis, IN, USA 46202

To order additional books, buy in bulk, or order for corporate use, contact Nursing Knowledge International at 888.NKI.4YOU (888.654.4968/US and Canada) or +1.317.634.8171 (outside US and Canada).

To request a review copy for course adoption, e-mail solutions@nursingknowledge.org or call 888.NKI.4YOU (888.654.4968/US and Canada) or +1.317.634.8171 (outside US and Canada).

To request author information, or for speaker or other media requests, contact Marketing at 888.634.7575 (US and Canada) or +1.317.634.8171 (outside US and Canada).

ISBN: 9781937554637
EPUB ISBN: 9781937554644
PDF ISBN: 9781937554651
MOBI ISBN: 9781937554668

Library of Congress Cataloging-in-Publication Data

Cavalieri, R. Jennifer (Ruth Jennifer), 1957-
  Clinical research manual : practical tools and templates for managing clinical research / R. Jennifer Cavalieri, Mark E. Rupp.
     p. ; cm.
  Includes bibliographical references and index.
  ISBN 978-1-937554-63-7 (book : alk. paper) – ISBN 978-1-937554-64-4 (EPUB) – ISBN 978-1-937554-65-1 (PDF) – ISBN 978-1-937554-66-8 (MOBI)
  I. Rupp, Mark E. II. Sigma Theta Tau International. III. Title.
  [DNLM: 1. Biomedical Research. 2. Clinical Trials as Topic. 3. Research Design. W 20.5]
  R853.C55
  610.72'4–dc23
                          2013012882

First Printing, 2013

Publisher: Renee Wilmeth
Acquisitions Editor: Emily Hatch
Editorial Coordinator: Paula Jeffers
Cover Designer: Michael Tanamachi
Interior Design/Page Layout: Katy Bodenmiller

Principal Book Editor: Carla Hall
Development and Project Editor: Susan Zingraf
Copy Editor: Heather Wilcox
Proofreaders: Andrew Kimmel and Heather Wilcox
Indexer: Johnna Van Hoose Dinse

Dedication

We dedicate this book to our past, present, and future research subjects whose generous actions allow us to help push back the boundaries of medical and scientific ignorance.

Acknowledgments

Thanks...for the encouragement and feedback

    Jon Beck, BS, PharmD

    Cindy Cowardin RN, BSN, CCRP

    Beth La Fave, BSMT, MS

    Elizabeth R. Lyden, MS

    Michelle M. Paul, BSN, CRA

    Tara Scrogin, JD

Thanks...for the technical support

    Sue Beach, BA

Thanks...to my mentors

    Beth Furlong, PhD, JD, RN

    Eileen Wirth, PhD

    Carol Zuegner, PhD

    Ann Yager, BS, RT (R)(T)

About the Authors

R. Jennifer Cavalieri, BSN, RN, CCRC, CCRP, has been a research nurse for more than 20 years. Her experience includes coordinating clinical research trials sponsored by the pharmaceutical industry, federal agencies, and investigator-initiated trials. She has also worked as a dedicated subject recruiter and manager of a clinical trials office. She has a 10-year professional affiliation with her co-author and is currently working in the Infectious Diseases section at the University of Nebraska Medical Center. Ms. Cavalieri's research interests are in the areas of subject recruitment, clinical trial budgeting, and study operations. She has been a member of Sigma Theta Tau International, Iota Tau Chapter, since 1998.

Mark E. Rupp, MD, is professor and chief of Infectious Diseases and medical director of the Department of Infection Control and Epidemiology at the University of Nebraska Medical Center. His research experience includes leading numerous infectious disease bench and clinical trials as the principal investigator. Dr. Rupp is past president of the Society of Healthcare Epidemiology of America (SHEA) and has authored more than 100 peer-reviewed scientific papers. He was the medical director for a hospital-based clinical trials office and has served as an advisor for the CDC, FDA, NIH, and VA. Dr. Rupp's research interests are in the areas of staphylococcal disease, antibiotic resistance, and health care–associated infections. He is recognized for his clinical expertise and is a frequent lecturer at national and international meetings.

Table of Contents

About the Authors ix
Introduction xix

1   Introduction to Clinical Research Operations 1
    How to Get What You Need From This Book 2
    Research Fundamentals 3
    Key Regulatory Resources 5
    Study Types 6
        Case Reports/Case Studies 7
        Ecologic Studies 7
        Cross-Sectional Studies 8
        Case Control Studies 8
        Cohort Studies 8
        Quasi-Experimental Studies 9
        Randomized, Controlled Trials 9
    Study Design 10
    Funding Sources 12
    Effective Strategies for Working With
    Clinical Staff 13
    Key Take-Aways 16
    Suggested Reading 16
    References 16

2   Site Administration 17
    Research Roles and Responsibilities 18
        Some Essential Functions to Consider 18
        Working With Study Sponsors 19
        Research Personnel 19
        Compliance Considerations 24
        Finance: The View From an Administrative Level 24
        Standard Operating Procedures 25
        Research Property and Equipment 27

Research Supplies 30
Research Space 30
Managing Risk 31
Time-Management Strategies 32
Tips for Staying Sane 34
Key Take-Aways 35
Suggested Reading 35
References 35

3 Managing Financial Processes 37
Research Roles and Financial Responsibilities 38
The Research Finance Life Cycle 39
    The Feasibility Process 39
    Study Budgets 42
Leveraging Site Logistics to Overcome Budget Shortfalls 62
The Contract Process 66
Reconciling Payments 70
Assessing the Financial Outcomes of a Clinical Trial 71
Creating a Resource Network 72
"Holes in the Boat": Common Ways Sites Can Lose Focus and Dollars 73
Key Take-Aways 75
Suggested Reading 76
References 76

4 Managing Regulatory Activities and Documents 77
Research Roles and Regulatory Responsibilities 78
Delegation of Tasks 79
Clinical Trial Documents 80
Regulatory Oversight for Research Activities 81
Research and Clinical Laboratories 85
Organizing Regulatory Documents 87
Audits and Inspections 90

   Fraud and Misconduct 91
    Routine Study Monitoring 93
  Roaming and Credentialing Activities 95
  Key Take-Aways 96
  Suggested Reading 97
  References 97

5 Working With Institutional Review Boards (Ethics Committees) 99
  Research Roles and Responsibilities 100
  Get to Know Your IRB 100
  The IRB Process 100
   New Study Approvals 101
   IRB Documents 108
  IRB Policies 118
  Building a Relationship With Your IRB 119
  Miscellaneous Activities and Details 121
  Key Take-Aways 121
  Suggested Reading 122
  References 122

6 Managing Clinical Trial Activities and Processes 123
  Research Roles and Responsibilities 124
  Organizing Workflow 125
  Clinical Workflow 125
   Starting Up a New Study 126
   Site Evaluation Visit Day 126
   Investigator Meetings 129
   Regulatory Start-Up 133
   Subject Recruitment 133
   Patient Tips and Strategies 136
   Study Visit Tips 136
   Specimen Collection 142

        Administration of Study Medication 146
        Activities After the Study Visit 146
    Organizing the Administrative/Clerical Workflow 148
        Documentation and Reports 153
        Financial Reports 154
        Progress Reports 155
        Correspondence 155
        Research Team Communication 156
        Weekly Updates 158
    Study Closeout 159
    Key Take-Aways 160
    Suggested Reading 161
    References 161

7 Managing Data and Research Records 163
    Research Roles and Responsibilities 164
    Data 164
        Data Integrity 164
        Data Ownership 166
        Retention of Study Data 166
    Documentation 167
        Source Documents 167
        Case Report Forms 169
        Note to File 169
        Source Document Binder 170
    Creating Documentation Tools 172
    Strategies for Organization 175
        Communication 175
        Intermediate Filing 176
        Reusable Supplies 177
    Key Take-Aways 177
    Suggested Reading 177

8	Professional Development	179
	Next Steps	180
	Journal Clubs	180
	Research Posters	182
	Professional Associations	183
	Certification	183
	Continuing Education	184
	Pop Quiz	185
	Closing Remarks	186
	Key Take-Aways	186
	Suggested Reading	186
	Appendix A	187
	Appendix B	193
	Index	255

Table of Forms: Your Research Tool Box

FORM/TABLE	PAGE	CHAPT.	TITLE	FORM TYPE	PURPOSE
1.1, 6.5	15, 157	1	Clinical Trial Summary	Word-text	communication
2.1	20	2	Key Contacts List	Word-text	communication
3.1	41	3	Financial Document Binder Table of Contents	Word-text	reminder list for document organization
3.1	42	3	Study Budget	EXCEL	financial workbook
3.2, 6.4	43, 154	3	Schedule of Events (SOE)	EXCEL	protocol reference
3.5	49	3	Budget Workbook	EXCEL	expense review and notes on calculations
3.6	50	3	Effort Log options	EXCEL	tracking hours
3.7	56	3	Stipend Tracker	EXCEL	tracking stipend payments
3.8	57	3	Labor Worksheet	EXCEL	detailed calculation of labor hours
3.9	59	3	Tests and Laboratory Tests	EXCEL	detailed calculation of test costs
3.10	60	3	Investigational Pharmacy Services	EXCEL	detailed calculation of pharmacy service fees
3.11	70	3	Sponsor Payment Remittance Detail	EXCEL	sponsor payment detail
3.12	71	3	Payment Reconciliation Log	EXCEL	tracking payments
3.13	72	3	Financial Worksheet	EXCEL	high level reconciliation of expenses and revenue
4.1, 7.1	80, 165	4	Site Staff Task Delegation Log	Word-text	detailed listing of study roles and responsibilities
4.2	88	4	Regulatory Document Binder Table of Contents	Word-text	reminder list for document organization
4.3, 6.2	95, 129	4	Site Visit Log	Word-text	documentation tool for site visits and visitors
5.1	106	5	Checklist for Regulatory Documents	EXCEL	documentation tool for regulatory submissions
5.2	108	5	Subject Demographic Tracker	Word-text	documentation tool
5.3	111	5	Billing Tracker for Grant Charges	EXCEL	documentation tool

FORM/ TABLE	PAGE	CHAPT.	TITLE	FORM TYPE	PURPOSE
5.4	113	5	Master Subject Log	Word-text	documentation tool
5.5, 7.5	114, 174	5	Informed Consent Documentation Tool	Word-text	documentation tool
5.6	117	5	SAE Summary Form	Word-text	documentation tool
6.1	128	6	Site Evaluation Visit	Word-text	reminder items for site visit w/agenda
6.2, 4.3	129, 95	6	Site Visit Log	Word-text	see 4.3
6.3	152	6	Study Reminder Checklist	Word-text	reminder list for activity organization
6.4, 3.2	154, 43	6	Schedule of Events (SOE)	EXCEL	protocol activities reference
6.5, 1.1	157, 15	6	Clinical Trial Summary	Word-text	communication
6.6	159	6	Weekly Report	Word-text	reminder items for meeting
7.1, 4.1	165, 80	7	Site Staff Delegation Log	Word-text	detailed listing of study roles and responsibilities
7.2	168	7	Screening Visit Checklist	Word-text	reminder items for study visits
7.3	170	7	Source Document Binder Contents	Word-text	reminder list for document organization
7.4	173	7	Investigational Drug Talking Points	Word-text	reminder list for study visit education
7.5, 5.5	174, 114	7	Informed Consent Documentation Tool	Word-text	documentation tool
8.1	181	8	Journal Article Summary Sheet	Word-text	reminder and documentation tool

---

See Appendix B (pages 193–254) for blank forms and examples of using and modifying the forms presented throughout the book.

Introduction

One of the main reasons why we find clinical trial research to be so rewarding is that it provides a wide array of intellectual challenges, and each trial offers the opportunity to discover answers to real-world research questions. This book is the result of more than 20 years of our experience spent working on dozens of trials. This book is for professionals interested in clinical research, whether they are formulating an investigator-initiated project, managing the clinical trial process, or working within a trial in any role.

This book is divided into key topic areas of research, and each chapter provides a framework and understanding of a fundamental area of a clinical trial. This book is intended to offer practical advice and covers who the key players are, the inner workings of the processes, everyday examples, and related references.

Here are some examples of key questions and misconceptions in research and how this book provides explanations and examples:

- "How do I objectively assess whether a trial is feasible?" Chapter 3 discusses clinical trial budgeting and contracting as well as the importance of understanding site expenses. Chapter 6 addresses subject recruitment and study visit logistics. All these components contribute to the feasibility decision.

- "What are my risks if I take on a clinical trial, and could they be mitigated?" Chapter 2 covers some common risks faced by investigators, strategies for risk mitigation, and contingency planning.

- "How do I leverage existing resources to reach my study goals?" Chapter 3 provides an example of how the investigator leveraged existing resources to optimize logistics and successfully conducted a modestly funded clinical trial.

- "I will definitely meet the enrollment goal for this clinical trial for pneumonia patients because I admit two or three potential subjects to the ICU every week." Confidence is good but can be dangerous if it leads to assumptions of instant success with study recruitment.

Chapter 3 discusses how the authors conduct a feasibility assessment and Chapter 6 covers the importance of planning and managing the recruitment process.

- "How can I efficiently navigate the regulatory approval processes at my research site?" Chapters 4 and 5 provide an overview and some practical tips for working with IRBs.

- "I am applying for this position as a research coordinator because I would like to have a nice quiet job." Chapter 1 presents foundational information about the importance, complexity, and magnitude of the regulatory landscape. Chapters 3 through 7 look closely at the everyday responsibilities of research personnel. Successful research professionals are skilled at critical thinking, problem solving, juggling priorities, and multitasking.

Some things you might not have realized:

- Research teams can comprise a wide variety of personnel who make specialized contributions. Generalized comments from their perspectives are included in Chapter 2.

- Are you familiar with the ALCOA principles for documentation? Chapter 7 discusses these and other data-related tips.

- Shipping biological samples requires compliance with the study protocol, your institution's policies, and national and international authorities. Chapter 6 presents an overview of some of the regulatory entities or agencies involved in this process as well as some tips for working with research specimens. What you don't know *can* hurt you.

This guidebook has been written for a wide variety of persons involved in clinical research, including those who are just beginning their work in research, such as the new research coordinator who asks, "Can I just follow you around for a couple of days to see how this is done?" It is also for those already in clinical research who find that they are spending most of their time correcting problems and are looking for ideas about how to proactively improve their research operations. Curious specialists, such as investigational pharmacists, statisticians, and financial administrators, have asked us about what happens "upstream" and "downstream" from the part of the study activities that they are directly involved in, so they should find this monograph interesting. Study sponsors who work with the high-level logistics of protocol development and application of the protocol across multiple sites and their onsite study monitors usually have a very limited view of the everyday research-site logistics, and we hope that this book will broaden their perspective.

Chapter 1
Introduction to Clinical Research Operations

Perhaps you have opened this book because you have questions about clinical research—not theory or regulatory questions, but everyday questions about the details and intricate aspects of conducting research, such as "How do I know which regulations are the most important ones to start learning, and how can I find them?" or "How do I objectively assess whether a trial is feasible?" or "What are the risks for starting a new clinical trial, and how can I mitigate those risks?" or "How do I leverage the existing resources at my site and reach my study goals?" These are the right questions to be asking whether you are new to research or trying to optimize an existing research program. The biggest challenge facing investigators and their research staff can be figuring out how to "do" the study activities and how to "do" them as efficiently as possible.

Research professionals may discuss operational details in sidebar conversations or when orienting or teaching new employees, but published discussions of research operations are often limited to brief summaries of study methods. This book provides examples of the activities involved in clinical trial operations at an academic research site.

There are formal avenues for learning about research conduct. Many college and university programs introduce research concepts at the undergraduate level. Graduate programs teach research theory, and students are involved in research projects. In the clinical practice setting, seasoned investigators may mentor new investigators. Larger research enterprises may have enough staff and resources to provide formal orientation and assign seasoned staff to teach and coach new employees. For many, learning the operational details around conducting research is a matter of trial and error.

This book was written for research professionals with or without formal training and provides information about the everyday logistics involved in performing clinical research trials. Most of the information in the book focuses on the activities done between the time an abstract is developed and the final analysis of the study data. We have included some information about administrative infrastructure and the contracting and billing processes. It is our hope that the examples in this book will serve as a springboard for use with your own clinical trials work.

How to Get What You Need From This Book

This book is not a novel, and our approach to presenting the research concepts in this book is not linear. So if you have an urgent challenge—for example, you learn about a funding opportunity for a research study or you have accepted a new position as a research coordinator—you may choose to start reading a certain chapter for what you need to know right now. We have considered what content to include in this book in order to help you see that while, for example, you may be concerned about getting Institutional

Review Board (IRB) approval for your study and go directly to Chapter 5 for information, there are then other regulatory matters for you to consider that are identified in Chapter 4.

In Chapter 1 we introduce some key research definitions, concepts, and roles. In each chapter throughout the book, we focus on an operational research topic and include discussion about the related research roles and responsibilities. We also provide examples of templates, forms, and workbooks to use that are helpful for tracking and maintaining key study information, and the Appendix includes blank versions that can be copied and used. Keep in mind that this book is providing some general information and examples for you to consider. Your site will probably have operational differences. In our experience, the operations, roles, and responsibilities have varied at each research site where we have worked. Examples in this book are taken from real-life experiences to help you understand the concepts we are presenting.

It is important to recognize that clinical research is dynamic, and what was acceptable practice yesterday or at another institution or for another study may not be universally applicable or approved. As a research professional, we are all expected to use our professional judgment for what is appropriate and to work under the guidance of the study sponsor and institutional review board (IRB). This is an "idea" book, and we hope it will be useful to you as such.

Research Fundamentals

We can start with some common terms used in research. These terms, and many more, can also be found in the glossary on the National Institutes of Health website, www.nih.gov, which is listed in the Suggested Reading section at the end of this chapter.

A *clinical trial* is "a research study using human subjects to evaluate the effect of interventions or exposures on biomedical or health-related outcomes. Two types of clinical studies are interventional studies (or clinical trials) and observational studies."

A *principal investigator (PI)* is the person responsible for the scientific and technical direction for the entire study. Additional investigators may be involved in a study, and they may be referred to as *secondary investigators*.

Additional members of a research team may include financial administrators, research coordinators and assistants, investigational pharmacists, dieticians, laboratory specialists, and statisticians. While some clinical research teams have a large number of personnel involved, it is not uncommon for team members to have multiple roles. For example, the research coordinator may also have administrative responsibilities.

A *research coordinator* is usually responsible for the daily clinical trial activities that include supporting recruitment, study visit activities, and documentation. Research coordinators may be nurses, medical technologists, or respiratory therapists.

People who participate in a clinical trial are *human subjects* or *participants*.

The *research site* refers to the location where the research is conducted. An academic research center is an institution where patients receive medical care and clinical trials are conducted. The investigators are medical providers caring for hospitalized and clinic patients. These patients may consent to participate in the research.

A *protocol* is a written plan that describes the clinical-trial activities. The primary elements of a protocol are sections on the scientific background, the purpose and objectives of the study, a description of the study design, and the statistical plan.

The protocol for clinical research trials typically has a formal title that may include a description of the type of trial and what is going to be done—for example,

> "A PHASE 2, RANDOMIZED, DOUBLE-BLIND, PLACEBO-CONTROLLED, DOSE-RANGING STUDY TO ASSESS THE SAFETY AND EFFICACY OF XXX FOR PREVENTION OF YYY IN ADULTS PREVIOUSLY TREATED FOR ZZZ."

> **TIP**
>
> *Investigators and their staff may assign short, unique nicknames for each of their studies, such as "the dressing study" or "the bathing study," for convenience purposes.*
>
> *Generally speaking, it is probably best to avoid creating a nickname for a study that contains the industrial sponsor's name. It is not unusual for a site to work on multiple studies for an industrial sponsor over time, and using a sponsor-naming convention can lead to confusion.*

> **TIP**
>
> *Some strategies for learning research terminology include using trusted websites to look up definitions, or research personnel can check the research protocol for an appendix containing the definitions of the study terms and acronyms. A trusted website includes those from the federal government (e.g., NIH, CDC, etc.) or professional societies (e.g., American Cancer Society, Amercian Heart Association, Infectious Disease Society of America, etc.).*

Key Regulatory Resources

Research regulations can seem overwhelming when you begin in research. Two foundational sources of regulatory guidance are the Food and Drug Administration (FDA) website, www.fda.org, and the International Committee on Harmonisation (ICH) website, www.ich.org. These websites contain a wealth of information and guidance on research regulations and Good Clinical Practice (GCP).

The FDA regulations related to working with human subjects are available on its website, www.fda.gov. These are three of the key FDA regulations that clinical research personnel who are working with human subjects will need to understand:

- 21 CFR 11 (Title 21 of the Code of Federal Regulations Part 11) (U.S. Food and Drug Administration, 2012r) addresses electronic documentation and electronic signatures.

- 21 CFR 50 (Title 21 of the Code of Federal Regulations Part 50) (U.S. Food and Drug Administration, 2012l) addresses the protection of human subjects.

- 21 CFR 56 (Title 21 of the Code of Federal Regulations Part 56) (U.S. Food and Drug Administration, 2012m) addresses Institutional Review Boards (IRBs).

> **TIP**
>
> *These regulations can give the research professional a deeper appreciation of why certain policies and procedures are in place at the institutional level and a better understanding of where the IRB gains its authority and approach to research issues. (IRBs are covered in detail in Chapter 5.)*

Clinical trial regulations are discussed in further detail in Chapters 4 and 5.

Study Types

Many types of research studies are available. Understanding what they are, their advantages and disadvantages, and how they are commonly used can help researchers decide which study design type is best to answer their research questions and help the other research professionals better understand the processes and activities involved.

Case Reports/Case Studies

A case report or case study is a method of research where detailed consideration and intensive analysis is conducted on a particular patient's illness or a specific event. Although by nature they are anecdotal, at times they can be very important. An example of this type of report would be an index case of an infection due to a novel agent. The limitations are that case reports describe a small number of patients and may not be generalizable. This type of study has no comparison group, so no association or causality can be inferred. However, case reports are valuable for promoting the formulation of a hypothesis that can become the basis for a more rigorous study.

For example, a patient with an infection due to vancomycin-resistant enterococcus (VRE) is noted to have received vancomycin three times in the previous 6 months. Does vancomycin treatment cause or select for VRE? In addition, a series of cases can be described, and, if done with enough epidemiologic detail, a more rigorous hypothesis regarding causality can be formulated.

Ecologic Studies

Ecologic studies can be used to make a comparison of trends in a condition to possible contributing factors. It usually makes use of aggregate data or an existing database. An example would be trends in cigarette smoking compared with trends in cardiac disease.

The advantages of this type of study are that it is easy and quick to perform and can therefore provide early support for a hypothesis. The disadvantage is that it does not distinguish between different hypotheses that can be consistent with the data. Generally, ecologic studies do not include patient-level data. For example, the rate of cardiac disease may correlate with the rate of cigarette smoking, but the database does not indicate whether patients with cardiac disease smoked cigarettes.

Cross-Sectional Studies

Cross-sectional studies, also called point prevalence studies, are surveys of a sample population to determine whether a particular risk factor is present. A point prevalence study might establish how many patients who have a urinary catheter in place also have bacteriuria. The advantage is that these studies are relatively easy to perform. Because the assessment is performed at a fixed point, it does not require follow-up of the study population. The disadvantage is that a point prevalence study does not capture elapsed time or transition. For example, this type of study does not provide for follow-up with patients with urinary catheters to see how many develop bacteriuria or symptomatic urinary tract infections.

Case Control Studies

Case control studies are conducted to determine whether there is an association between a risk factor and an outcome. A characteristic feature is that subjects are enrolled as cases or controls based on the presence or absence of a specific outcome. The two groups are compared to assess the presence of a proposed risk factor. To optimize the ability to examine specific risk factors, the cases and controls should be matched as evenly as possible.

The advantage of this type of study is that the investigator can enroll all defined cases, making it an attractive option when the outcome is rare. Multiple risk factors can be evaluated, provided that the investigator thinks of the various factors. The disadvantages of this type of study are that they are retrospective and subject to various types of bias. The investigator must be very careful when defining cases and controls that are representative of the population.

Cohort Studies

In cohort studies, subjects are enrolled based on the presence or absence of an exposure instead of the presence of an outcome. They can be prospective, concurrent, retrospective, nonconcurrent, or database studies. The advantages are a better assessment of causality and the investigator's ability to study multiple outcomes from a single risk or exposure. The disadvantages are that they are costly and can have time constraints. If the outcome is rare, a large cohort may be needed. These studies are also observational and therefore subject to bias.

Quasi-Experimental Studies

Quasi-experimental studies are nonrandomized, pre-, and post-intervention studies. They are often employed in outbreak situations or quality improvement interventions by "making a change and seeing what happens." The advantage to a quasi-experimental study is that it can be performed when ethical considerations preclude performing a randomized trial. They can be done in situations where immediate action is required, and they are logistically easier than performing a randomized trial involving a control population.

The disadvantages to quasi-experimental studies are that it is difficult to control for confounding variables, there is a poor link to causality, and they may be subject to a "regression to the mean" phenomenon in which occurrence of an outcome or disease may moderate spontaneously (e.g., outbreaks tend to diminish over time). The Latin phrase "*post hoc ergo propter hoc*," which means "after this therefore because of this," may not hold true. In other words, just because an intervention is introduced is no guarantee that a change that is observed is due to the intervention. In recent years, the design of quasi-experimental studies has often been enhanced by inclusion of crossover interventions and washout periods.

Randomized, Controlled Trials

Randomized, controlled trials (RCTs) are prospective, and the randomization, if done effectively, limits bias. Ideally, subjects are assigned to intervention or control groups in a blinded fashion. RCTs are experimental rather than observational and are designed to test the effect of a planned intervention. Determination of the size of the trial (number of subjects in each group) is critical and depends on the incidence of the outcome measure in the control population as well as the effectiveness of the intervention.

This type of study design is the most convincing demonstration of causality. The disadvantage to RCTs is usually cost and logistical considerations. At times, ethical considerations are quite thorny, such as whether a placebo should be utilized. Also, RCTs can be subject to confounding.

Study Design

Although it is not within the scope of this book to delve extensively into research study design, statistical methods, or analysis of the literature, a basic understanding of study design and how to evaluate a study report is invaluable for the well-prepared research professional. A thorough understanding of these topics is required before proposing an investigator-initiated study.

> **TIP**
>
> *In analyzing a study or study report, it is important to consider the framework of the study, which includes the study design, assignment of subjects, assessment of outcome, analysis of results, and, finally, the interpretation and extrapolation of the results.*

Study design involves the hypothesis, study population, sample size, and statistical power of a study. The *hypothesis*, or the research question, drives the study design.

The *study population* is proscribed by the inclusion and exclusion criteria and greatly affects the extrapolation of findings to other settings. The *sample size*, or the number of subjects or observations, needs to be large enough to demonstrate statistical significance if the hypothesis is true. It is not necessary to be a biostatistician to be a successful clinical researcher, but access to expert biostatistical advice is crucial in the design and analysis of all but the simplest studies.

Assignment is the method by which subjects are assigned to study and control groups. The goal is to select groups as similar as possible except for the presence or absence of a condition, exposure, or intervention. In well-performed prospective trials, randomization and masking should limit most types of bias. *Masking*, or blinding, is the process by which the results of the randomization of subjects to the intervention or control group are concealed from the study participants, the investigator and research personnel, or both. However, even when studies do not have bias, they can suffer from *confounding variables*.

Assessment involves defining the *endpoints*, or outcomes. These endpoints may be primary or secondary and need to be appropriate or relevant to the study question. They should also be unambiguous, free from error, and objective. The endpoint definitions should be precise to prevent intra-observer error. The endpoint assessment should be complete, with all subjects assessed with an equal intensity of observations. Preferably, the endpoints should be unaffected by the measurement process.

The *analysis* of results involves estimation of the strength of the association and any adjustment for potential confounding variables. The interpretation of results, or *conclusion*, should be supported by the data. When evaluating a study report, the reader should ask whether a statistically significant cause-and-effect association is demonstrated or whether a dose-response is noted. What has the investigator learned from the study that can be extrapolated to individuals outside the study? Although it is appropriate to speculate when discussing the results, it is important for investigators to not overreach in their conclusions. Astute readers will be dismayed at how often a conclusion of a study is overstated and not directly supported by the data derived from the study.

The terms *bias* and *confounding* have been used above. It is important for researchers to have an understanding of what these terms mean. *Bias* is a systematic error that results from errors in study design or conduct. In other words, the study produces an incorrect conclusion. Errors of bias cannot be overcome by adjustment and analysis. Confounding, on the other hand, can be adjusted by statistical techniques if it is recognized. *Confounding* has been defined as a "mixing" of effects, or a distortion of the outcome measurement caused by the presence of an extraneous factor.

A broad category of bias is selection or sampling bias. For example, if a study relies upon subjects to step forward and volunteer, there is a strong chance that individuals who volunteer are not representative of the general population. Another example would be the "man on the street" interview. Clearly, the subjects who will be sampled will be strongly affected by where the interview takes place (e.g., inner-city ghetto vs. affluent shopping center) and will likely exclude persons who are not ambulatory (e.g., chronically ill). These types of errors in study design or conduct cannot be corrected by statistical methods.

Confounding can occur in even very well-designed and appropriately conducted studies. For example, despite blinded randomization, at the time of data analysis, it is observed in a study examining the possible impact of a new antibiotic for treatment of pneumonia that substantially more patients with underlying smoking and COPD were enrolled in the control arm of the study. Thus, initially it is unclear whether the new antibiotic is better or whether the control population has a confounding variable that impacts the outcome. However, through statistical methods, the presence of smoking and COPD can be taken into account, and a valid conclusion can be reached.

From the above example, it should be evident to the reader that a larger, adequately powered study will be less likely to have the type of confounding illustrated than a smaller, less well-designed trial.

Funding Sources

Clinical trials can also be defined by how they are developed and funded. *Investigator-initiated trials* and *federally funded trials* begin with the investigator's idea and protocol design. Many industrial studies are funded by the pharmaceutical industry or device manufacturers, and in most cases the investigators are not involved in the protocol development, nor do they have any financial relationship with the investigational product or device or rights to intellectual property.

> **TIP**
>
> *If any member of the research team has a relationship with the study sponsor—for example, as a paid consultant—this information must be disclosed. All research personnel should be familiar with and comply with their institutions' conflict-of-interest policies.*

Effective Strategies for Working With Clinical Staff

Research personnel should recognize that there are similarities and differences in research and clinical priorities. But the common ground for research and clinical professionals is patient safety. Clinical practice is treatment oriented and follows clinical standards. Research professionals must not deviate from the protocol that has been created to answer a specific research question. Effective strategies for working with clinical staff to keep everyone on track with the goals of a study are:

- Identify the clinical stakeholders at the start of a new study, such as medical providers, clinical caregivers, and ancillary personnel in the pharmacy or laboratory.

- Meet with members of the clinical leadership teams during the study planning period. Inform them of the clinical trial's purpose and what the research team will be doing in their areas.

- Make the request for research-related support from clinical caregivers during the planning period. Clinical personnel will want to know about the study time line and projected volume of subjects and, when the time comes, the results of the study.

On an everyday basis, professional research behavior on an inpatient hospital unit or in the clinic includes providing the clinical caregivers with research updates and asking them for clinical updates. This type of communication promotes the safety of the patient/research subject, as each party—the caregiver and the research professional—has valuable patient information. A useful tool to support this communication from the beginning is shown in Form 1.1, Clinical Trial Summary, which contains essential study information and research contact information. (Be sure to document the clinical trial in the patient's medical record according to your institution's policy.)

The Clinical Trial Summary can be posted in the record or given to bedside clinical personnel to efficiently transfer basic information about the study to the subject's caregivers. Form 1.1 is representative of a Clinical Trial Summary recently used in an inpatient clinical trial.

EXAMPLE

A principal investigator (PI) wanted to conduct an investigator-initiated study in the ICU. By holding a planning meeting with the nurse manager of the unit, the PI was able to explain the purpose of the study, find common ground on the benefits of using the study outcomes for quality improvement in ICU activities, and clarify the role of the research nurse coordinator and how the coordinator would work collaboratively with the clinical staff, interact with the ICU patients, and collect the study data. The PI and the nurse manager negotiated a study start time to minimize any potential conflicts with the unit-based activities. The PI presented the study results within 1 month of the completion of the study. This rapid-cycle feedback gave the clinical staff evidence-based results and was a positive reinforcement to the clinical personnel of the value of conducting research.

FORM 1.1 Clinical Trial Summary

	CLINICAL TRIAL SUMMARY
Title of Trial	*Effectiveness of chlorhexidine gluconate (CHG) general skin cleansing in reducing the occurrence of catheter-associated bloodstream infections and the transmission and/or infection rate due to multi-drug resistant organisms in hospitalized patients.*
IRB Number/Approval	*xxx*
Name of Trial	*CHG Bathing Study*
Investigator	*Mark E. Rupp, M.D.*
Coodinator	Name: *Jen Cavalieri, BSN, RN, CCRC, CCRP* **Telephone:** *(111)222-3456* **Pager:** *(444)555-6789*
Purpose of Study	*The purpose of this study is to determine the effect of daily bathing with a dilute solution of chlorhexidine gluconate on the rate of intravascular catheterassociated infections and the reate of acquisition/ transmission or infection due to specific micro-organisms.*
Enrollment Goal	*All patients hospitalized with the exception of neonates and new-born nursery patients.*
Study Duration	**Start:** *16 February 09* **End:** *August 2011*
Procedures	1. Chlorhexidine (CHG) bathing will be introduced first to patients in the ICU areas. For the first six months, CHG bathing will be done on Mondays-Wednesdays-Fridays. After the initial six month period, CHG bathing frequency will be increase to daily. 2. At the three month milestone, CHG bathing will be introduced to the remainder of patients in the hospital on a Monday-Wednesday-Friday schedule. After six months, the CHG bathing frequency will increased to daily. 3. The Investigational Product is stocked in the supply machines on each unit. Staff will remove product for their patients on a daily basis. There is no patient charge 4. Patients and parents of pediatric patients are advised to use the CHG with bathing/showering applying the product from the neck down. 5. Research staff will be collecting monthly census and bottle usage data 6. Patients may decline to bathe with Hibiclens. 7. Adverse events will be monitored by notifications from the clinical staff and/or the hospital incident reporting system.
Possible Risks	• Extensively used for several decades • Dermatologic reactions- no evidence of absorption, low potential for reactions • Case reports of hypersensitivity, anaphylaxis,, ototoxicity, corneal injury are rare

QUESTIONS? Jen Cavalieri Research Nurse Coordinator
Phone here - Pager here Email: here

Key Take-Aways

- Learning about research fundamentals and operations is an ongoing process.

- Being familiar with and following regulations is essential in all research studies and trials.

- Always consider the responsibilities and priorities of clinical staff.

Suggested Reading

Chan et al. SPIRIT 2013 statement: Defining standard protocol items for clinical trials. Annals of Internal Medicine. Jan. 2013. Retrieved from http://annals.org/article.aspx?articleid=1556168

Fedor, C. (2006). Responsible research: A guide for coordinators. London: Remedica Pub Ltd.

National Institutes of Health. www.nih.gov

References

National Institutes of Health, Office of Extramural Research. (2012, December). Glossary & acronym list. Retrieved from http://grants.nih.gov/grants/glossary.htm#A27

U.S. Food and Drug Administration. (2012b, April 1). CFR – Code of Federal Regulations Title 21, Chapter 1, Subchapter A, Part 56 Institutional Review Boards. Retrieved from http://www.accessdata.fda.gov/scripts/cdrh/cfdocs/cfcfr/cfrsearch.cfm?cfrpart=56

U.S. Food and Drug Administration. (2012e, April 1). CFR – Code of Federal Regulations Title 21, Chapter 1, Subchapter A, Part 11 Electronic Records; Electronic Signatures. Retrieved from http://www.accessdata.fda.gov/scripts/cdrh/cfdocs/cfcfr/CFRSearch.cfm?CFRPart=11&showFR=1&subpartNode=21:1.0.1.1.7.3

U.S. Food and Drug Administration. (2012l, April 1). CFR – Code of Federal Regulations Title 21, Chapter 1, Subchapter A, Part 50 Protection of Human Subjects. Retrieved from http://www.accessdata.fda.gov/scripts/cdrh/cfdocs/cfcfr/cfrsearch.cfm?cfrpart=50

U.S. Food and Drug Administration. (2012m, April 1). CFR – Code of Federal Regulations Title 21, Chapter 1, Subchapter D, Part 314 Applications for FDA Approval to Market a New Drug. Retrieved from http://www.accessdata.fda.gov/scripts/cdrh/cfdocs/cfcfr/cfrsearch.cfm?cfrpart=314

U.S. Food and Drug Administration. (2012r, April 1). CFR – Code of Federal Regulations Title 21, Chapter 1, Subchapter A, Part 11 Electronic Records; Electronic Signatures, Subpart C Electronic Signatures. Retrieved from http://www.accessdata.fda.gov/scripts/cdrh/cfdocs/cfCFR/CFRSearch.cfm?fr=11.100

Chapter 2
Site Administration

Administrative processes at your research site are the infrastructure needed to support all your study endeavors. While we may take some of these things for granted or triage them as a lower priority to be done "someday," they will be the first things needed when an auditor knocks on the door or a crisis, such as absent staff, occurs.

One strategy is for you to quickly skim through the ideas in this chapter. If you can identify the biggest weaknesses at your research site, carve out some time daily or weekly to get some fundamentals in place, and then steadily progress on developing these processes, you will quickly have the essentials in place. This chapter provides you with ideas for setting up some key administrative processes, documents, and contingency plans.

Research Roles and Responsibilities

A variety of research professionals are involved in the administrative processes.

A research *investigator* is responsible for all aspects of conducting the study, which includes administrative duties. When a clinical trial has multiple investigators involved, a *principal investigator* (PI) will lead the entire research team.

Investigators may have administrative personnel within the infrastructure of their organization. Their research specific functions may include processing payroll, processing the sponsor's contract documents, and monitoring the financial accounts for grants.

Study *sponsors* are responsible for selecting investigators, providing the study protocol and training for investigators and their research staff, providing oversight for protocol compliance by using representatives (called study monitors), and working with the U.S. Food and Drug Administration (FDA) on the investigational drug or device processes, depending on the study type. They are also responsible for formally reporting serious adverse events and quality control activities (U.S. Food and Drug Administration, 2012j).

Research coordinators are responsible for supporting the day-to-day clinical trial activities, which includes tracking the sponsor and site stakeholders, research efforts, and study subject visits. Research coordinators who are involved with clinical trials involving human subjects are often nurses, medical technologists, or respiratory therapists.

Some Essential Functions to Consider

Administrative duties in research may include working with study sponsors, supervising research personnel, supporting regulatory compliance, maintaining financial records, establishing standard operating procedures (SOP), and acquiring physical materials, such as property, equipment, supplies, and space. All these functions are similar to common business practices in other professions. Just because we work in a clinical world does not mean there are limited choices for business activities.

One option for improving these processes is to look at business strategies and systems and identify practices to adopt in order to make your own administrative processes more efficient. Networking with business colleagues and evaluating ways to best manage teams is one way to eliminate inefficiencies and build on strengths.

Working With Study Sponsors

Study sponsors may have their own employees perform their study activities, or they may outsource selected tasks to specialized companies called *contract research organizations* (CROs). The sponsor remains ultimately responsible for all the study activities, but the CRO may be directly supporting the contracting, monitoring, or laboratory testing.

Creating a list of study stakeholders, see Form 2.1, Key Contacts List, can help clarify and keep the names, roles, and contact information of the people on both the sponsor/CRO and site sides readily available. The sooner this list is made available, the sooner it can help the communication process, and it can always be updated as needed.

For federally funded and industry-sponsored trials, the sponsor's representative, or study monitor, will regularly visit the study sites to review the regulatory files, study records, and investigational pharmacy for protocol compliance. This monitoring is necessary to ensure protocol compliance and the safety and rights of research subjects and to verify the quality and integrity of the data being collected.

Research Personnel

The investigator may delegate the daily business functions for managing research personnel to an administrator or manager, as the "people" part of the research team activities can be very time consuming. These activities may include scheduling, processing payroll, maintaining personnel files, and conducting performance appraisals.

Administrative management of research employees includes maintaining documentation of their training, certifications, competencies, and performance evaluations.

FORM 2.1 Key Contacts List (Word document form)

Study Name	
Study Site Number	
Sponsor	**Principal Investigator**
Name	Name
Address	Address
	Phone
Medical Monitor	Fax
Name	
Phone	**Secondary Investigator**
Email	Name
	Address
Sponsor Project Manager	Phone
Name	Fax
Phone	
Email	**Research Nurse Coordinator**
	Name
CRO	Phone
Name	Email
Phone	
	Lead Study Coordinator
Lead CRA	Name
Name of Study Monitor	Address
Phone	Phone
Email	Fax
CRO Regulatory	**Investigational Pharmacist**
Name of Regulatory Specialist	Name
Phone	Address
Email	Phone
	Fax
Central Laboratory	
Name of company outpatient	**Specialty Clinical Area** (such as echo lab, clinic, or microbiology bench)
Contact Person	Name
Office Phone	Phone
Email	

> **TIP**
>
> *Files for research professionals could contain copies of the job description; licenses; certifications, such as those for ethics training and hazardous shipping; and institutional competencies for infection control, blood-borne pathogen training, and use of personal protective equipment. In addition, copies of requests for time off and special recognitions can be kept in this file. Copies of performance appraisals and annual goals are also useful references to be kept in this file.*

An administrator might not know what the required research competencies are, what they specifically cover, or how often they need to be renewed. The administrator should check the institution's policies and can also work with research staff to learn what the relevant competencies are. He or she can create the staff and new employee orientation instructions and simple tracking spreadsheets.

All research professionals have a personal responsibility to maintain their professional documents. One can maintain one's own folder so that essential licensing, competency, and certifications are always readily available. Another idea is to maintain documentation at both home and work offices. Simply telling staff to maintain their own documents without some administrative oversight runs the risk of noncompliance that has repercussions for the staff member, the PI, and the institution. For example, lapsed licenses, shipping certifications, or ethics training can violate state law, jeopardize public safety, or hold up the internal study-approval processes.

> **TIP**
>
> *At academic medical centers, a curriculum vitae (CV) is the equivalent of a business résumé. A CV usually contains the person's contact information, academic rank, education, and experience. All presentations, publications, and awards are listed in detail. A biosketch is an abbreviated form of a CV that is commonly used as an attachment for federal grant applications.*

Research personnel often work on multidisciplinary teams. Members of the research team are chosen because of their specialized knowledge to perform certain study-related tasks. There may be a variety of perspectives on the tasks, priorities, and support needed to accomplish their assignments. So if you were to ask research professionals in a variety of different research and institutional positions what they would wish for to make their research activities easier, their answers might be:

Investigators:

- Adequate budgets
- Smooth site operations
- Well-designed protocols

Finance administrators:

- Clear, upfront instructions on the study payment process and detailed statements accompanying the sponsor payments
- Details about financial contacts and payment triggers
- A realistic estimate of the number of subjects that will be enrolled so that department budgets can be planned

Site contract personnel:

- Prompt completion of the necessary information and documents so that they can proceed with contract negotiation
- Understanding from sponsors and investigators that some things are beyond the control of the contract negotiator
- Not being used as a scapegoat when delays occur in getting a contract finalized

Research coordinators:

- Ability to network with other research coordinators internally and externally to gather tips and ideas about study logistics
- Additional background information about the medical condition being studied, including information on signs and symptoms, diagnostics, and prognosis

- User-friendly electronic case report form (eCRF) IT systems
- Movement of sponsors and monitors away from using FAX processes for sending in screening logs and ordering supplies to employing a web-based system that can also serve as a "real-time" newsletter and enrollment tally

Investigational pharmacists:

- Communication, communication, communication
- Friendly research coordinators, collegial respect and teamwork, and positive attitudes
- Reduction of redundant forms from sponsors

Clinical laboratory personnel:

- Clear instructions from investigators regarding what they want them to do or the types of tests required
- Friendly research personnel
- Research personnel who are conscientious and tidy when working in their lab space

Clinical caregivers:

- Communication about what research personnel are doing to their patients
- Instructions regarding what the PI wants them to do
- The study results

Biostatisticians:

- Inclusion in planning meetings
- Involvement in discussions about data collection
- Involvement in the development and formatting of the data spreadsheets in preparation for the analysis

This shows each team member's perspective, and, by communicating with colleagues, you may find opportunities to implement improvements to the work environment.

Compliance Considerations

A first step to understanding compliance-related matters at the research site is for the investigator and the administrator to identify the institution's compliance-related policies and procedures. These policies will be a useful resource to identify the key personnel and compliance areas. Research-related compliance may include special committees (beyond those for human subject and animal research), privacy policies, training requirements, grant billing policies, and reporting obligations and methods.

One example of these compliance policies is an institution's *Health Insurance Portability and Accountability* (HIPAA) compliance plan. The institution's policy may define related terms, identify key personnel serving in such roles as a privacy officer or security officer and their contact information, mandatory training requirements, and internal auditing processes.

Other key compliance policies are related to the use of and security measures for the institution's computer systems. These policies typically include guidance on computer use, electronic information security, user access and password security, incident reporting, and data storage and retrieval. For example, if computer systems need to have change control, a clear process that documents when changes are made to the information technology (IT) systems will be found in the compliance policies.

Finance: The View From an Administrative Level

Administrative records may contain the documents related to the financial aspects of each of the investigator's studies. Such items as sponsor contracts, conflict-of-interest information, records for all study expenses, and revenue payments are not customarily stored with the research data, and so these may be stored in administrative files.

Metrics can be determined for what to track in order to assess financial performance. The metrics for annual administrative reviews may include the total number of studies, subjects enrolled, and revenue and expenses. This information can be used to set quarterly and annual goals.

> **TIP**
>
> *The investigator's research finances may be a subset of the overall budgetary considerations. Individual study revenue and expenses are discussed in detail in Chapter 3.*

Standard Operating Procedures

SOPs are the investigator's plan for the research enterprise. An investigator's SOPs are descriptions of how the research activities are conducted at the site. SOPs should be based on FDA regulations and the International Conference on Harmonisation (ICH) guidelines for conducting clinical trials.

SOPs serve many purposes. They clarify how research activities are done at the investigator's site. They set expectations, and, because they define which and how things are to be done, they can be used to hold staff accountable. They also identify internal resources, such as policies and procedures.

> **TIP**
>
> *SOPs do not necessarily need to restate existing guidelines. They can be used to identify or reference internal and external resources, policies and procedures, and regulatory guidance.*

The investigator is ultimately responsible for the conduct of the research trials and for following the guidelines put forth in the institution's policies and his or her own SOPs. Investigators and administrators may also be involved in developing the content for SOPs.

Annual review of SOPs is prudent. Policies should truly reflect what is being done, not just fill pages in a binder stored on a shelf. The date of the latest version can be noted when a revised SOP is implemented, but the previous versions also need to be retained, as they reflect the SOPs in place during a particular time period. SOPs are valuable education and orientation tools.

SOP documents typically include several fundamental elements:

1) The name of the organization, the title of the SOP, the section of the reference manual where this particular SOP is located, when it was issued, when it was revised, and the number of pages. The investigator's institution may have templates or standard formats for SOP documents.

2) The purpose of the policy, clearly and simply stated. For example, a policy on delegation of authority may state that its purpose is to ensure that the leadership, chain of command, and contact information of the research group are clearly documented for research staff and the institution.

3) The scope of the policy identifying to whom the policy applies. For example, the policy on delegation of authority may apply to all research staff in the research group.

4) Responsibilities are clearly stated.

5) Any background information, such as references to FDA regulations or ICH guidelines, can be included.

6) A section describing procedures can provide instructions on what to do and whom to notify. For example, a policy on audits can include information about what to have ready for the inspector, whom to notify within the organization, research staff responsibilities, and follow-up activities. By creating a plan and SOP on how an audit would be handled, the investigator and site personnel will be better prepared in the event that an audit is necessary.

7) References and attachments are included as applicable.

8) The person(s) responsible for the creation and administration of the policy is clearly identified and has possibly signed and dated the documents.

So where should you start when faced with creating site SOPs, and how many SOPs do investigators need? One approach is to create a list of potential SOPs and then start to prioritize. For example, an SOP on delegation of authority to define the chain of command and an SOP on audits to prepare for when, not if, the research site is audited by internal or external examiners may be at the top of the list. The investigator and staff can create a list of additional topics and create a binder or electronic file with a section for each topic. As parts of the policy are drafted, reference materials are identified that can be saved in the binder or electronic folder until the investigator and staff are ready to finalize the policy.

By identifying a reasonable number of SOPs to begin with, time frames can be set for creating them—perhaps one a month. Within a year's time, a foundation of a dozen key SOPs will exist that can be built upon as needed.

Research Property and Equipment

Managing research property and equipment involves knowing what you have and maintaining security so the property is not lost.

> **TIP**
>
> *Signage stating the owner and contact information should be easily visible on all property and equipment.*

The administrative files can contain an inventory of all the research property, the owner manuals, documentation of calibration and maintenance, service agreements, and purchase receipts. This information is very useful in the event of equipment recalls and future purchasing decisions. Sometimes research personnel use equipment that is owned by other departments, such as the pharmacy or laboratory. Sharing particularly expensive or specialized equipment is practical, such as –70 degree freezers that cost thousands of dollars apiece. The clinical laboratory may have dozens or hundreds of pieces of equipment. If the research staff have research specimens processed in a refrigerated centrifuge or temporarily store specimens in a –70 degree freezer, documentation of the equipment number, copies of the calibration and equipment maintenance, and daily temperature logs are kept in the research regulatory binder. This documentation demonstrates that the specimens were processed and held according to protocol specifications, as temperature variations, or excursions, can affect specimen quality.

Research property includes furniture, equipment, and supplies. The investigator should differentiate between property that belongs to the investigator and the study sponsor. For example, the sponsor may provide an electrocardiogram machine for the site to use for research subject assessments during the trial but expect that it will be returned to the sponsor at the end of the study.

All equipment requires periodic inspection and calibration. Check whether your institution has personnel who can perform these routine services and repairs. For research purposes, documentation of the equipment tags and calibration records is usually subject to inspection. A photograph of the equipment can be placed in the file and may prove to be useful.

Refrigerators and freezers must be dedicated to the storage of food, drugs, medical specimens, or supplies. Dual usage is an unacceptable and unsafe practice (e.g., specimens should not be stored in the same refrigerator as medications or food). Documentation of temperature during supply shipments is standard practice. Temperature excursions require research staff to follow up and determine whether the unit contents are still usable. This monitoring can be as simple as using a high-low thermometer, manually recording the temperature, and keeping the temperature log sheets on file, or it can be as sophisticated as setting an alarm that is hardwired into the electrical and telephone systems to notify staff of temperature excursions.

At the end of the study, the study sponsor will typically provide directions regarding which study property and equipment are to be returned, kept by the investigators, or discarded.

SITE EXAMPLE

An SOP for research equipment may address:

- *Security, stating that "research property will be maintained in a secure environment with controlled access."*
- *Expectations for documentation, stating that "an inventory of property is maintained in a certain location and contains such items as user manuals, purchasing documentation, and photographs as appropriate." This documentation may reference institutional guidelines, such as "refrigerator/freezers will be monitored and maintained according to (institution name) policies and procedures," and attach the referenced policy.*
- *Purchasing authority, if not already stated in the delegation of authority SOP, stating that "purchases require approval from (name and title of person) with (institution name)." The title of the person with responsibility for conducting the purchasing process and maintaining the financial records is useful to include in the SOP. Research staff may provide technical advice and purchase justifications and may therefore also be included in the SOP.*

The SOP for research property belonging to study sponsors may include these additional statements:

- *The sponsor's property, which includes equipment and supplies, will be maintained in a secure environment with controlled access.*
- *Study-specific inventories will be maintained using the sponsor's documents and supplementary study-site documents as needed.*
- *Investigational drug supplies will be maintained and dispensed from (location). (Note: A description of the process for picking up the investigational product for study visit dosing can be described in the Investigational Pharmacy SOP.)*
- *All study documents, supplies, and equipment will be available during monitoring visits by sponsor/representatives.*

Research Supplies

It is important to keep an inventory of the supplies at the site. Surplus specimen cups, biohazard bags, and catheter hubs, for instance, may be useful for future studies. Supplies that belong to the study sponsor need to be returned unless the sponsor has given permission for the site to keep them. All supplies should be carefully inspected for expiration dates and discarded appropriately. Unneeded supplies may be donated to medical clinics for underserved or developing countries.

> **TIP**
>
> *If possible, store the supplies for each active study together to keep track of expiration dates, the quantity of collection kits, and requisition forms.*

Research Space

Research investigators and their personnel need office workspace. This space must have controlled access and the ability to secure documents and supplies, which usually necessitates computers and standard office equipment, such as telephones, scanners, and fax machines, and office furniture, such as desks and file cabinets. Subject study visits may occur on the inpatient units or in a clinic.

Research investigators need space where research monitors can come for their routine visits to review the research documents, and they need access to conference or meeting rooms for planning sessions or audits. Additional space considerations include accessible and secure storage space for supplies and records as well as short- and longer-term storage space for archiving study records.

> **TIP**
>
> *Office space at research sites is often at a premium. Research staff often have multiple reference binders open while they are working on computers. An L-shaped workspace is usually a helpful configuration.*

Managing Risk

The topic of research risk usually centers on subject safety. Although safety is a primary consideration, additional risks are frequently associated with clinical trials. As risks are identified, the investigator needs to decide whether they should be avoided, accepted, mitigated, or transferred.

In research, if the investigator feels the inclusion and exclusion criteria are so strict that the pool of potential subjects is not large enough to find eligible subjects, the investigator may forecast never reaching a financial break-even point and thus *avoid the risk* by not participating in the clinical trial.

Accepting risk means the investigator is taking no action to reduce the probability or impact of risk. If an investigator opens a study but is never able to enroll eligible subjects and then takes on another, similar trial, the investigator is accepting the risk that the same result may occur.

Examples of ways to *mitigate*, or lessen the impact of, a risk would be to conduct a feasibility assessment or to perform a retrospective chart review to check whether the investigator's patient population would meet the study inclusion or exclusion criteria. Another option for mitigating risk is to cross-train staff to perform a variety of study tasks.

Transferring the risk involves shifting responsibilities. For example, the sponsor may propose a budget with payments only for enrolled subjects, which is sometimes referred to as a "pay-for-performance" arrangement. By doing this, the sponsor has transferred the risk of low or no subject enrollment onto the site investigator.

Successful clinical trials rely on the investigator's ability to identify disruptors, or risks; forecast the probability that these will occur; assess their potential impact on study operations; and plan accordingly. Some examples of site risk include employee absences or turnover.

The first step is for the investigator to recognize that some things are beyond control and to work through potential solutions before a crisis is at hand. Employees miss work due to illness or accept other employment opportunities, sometimes people can act irrationally and harm others, or a variety of catastrophic weather-related events, such as a blizzard, hurricane, or man-made disaster, can occur at the investigator's institution or in the local region, halting research operations for days, months, or longer. The investigator needs to work through these possibilities and develop contingency plans based on the probability of occurrence and impact these events would have on the research operations.

The probability that an employee will occasionally be absent due to illness is relatively high. Some potential solutions that could be implemented include documenting tasks and processes in an SOP so that someone else can cover for a temporary absence or train a new employee. Another option is for research staff to work as a team. This structure broadens everyone's experience and promotes professional growth. The probability of severe weather or threats from irrational people halting research activities is probably lower. However, emergency preparedness with some contingency plans that include emergency communication, drills, and clarification of responsibilities during an internal or external disaster are necessary. Although these contingency plans may never need to be implemented, the modest amount of time spent preparing them can be time well spent.

Preparing some standardized documents, such as a brief study-specific summary for each of the investigator's trials, would be a useful tool for triaging during a disaster. In the event the investigator or the research coordinator is not readily available, any member of the investigator's research staff can take this document to members of the leadership team managing the disaster so they are able to triage based on the essential information in the reference. Having this information would put them in a better position to make decisions about subject safety and how to support or transition subjects off investigational drugs.

Time-Management Strategies

Organization and effective time management make workdays much more productive and pleasant. Here are some strategies to encourage efficiency:

- Be responsible for critical thinking and decision-making within the scope of your research role. Figure out what needs to be done rather than wait for someone to tell you what to do.

- Connect tasks with outcomes. Every task should clearly support a measureable and valuable result. Perfect source document checklists are useless if no subjects get enrolled into the study.
- Be prepared. Set up study visit materials a day in advance. Create a meeting file and put relevant items in it or make notes about items to discuss or bring to the meeting. Create a detailed agenda, placing highest-priority discussion items at the top of the list. Bring two copies to the meeting (one for you and one for the investigator) or e-mail the agenda before the meeting so the investigator can review it to prepare for the meeting.
- Focus on making interactions effective by routinely asking your investigator or research staff such questions as "What's your research priority today?" Offer them a status report. It is important to understand the status of projects in order to efficiently manage the trials.
- Be decisive.
- Keep copies of everything.
- Create binders or folders for clinical trials as soon as they start so all documentation and information stays together.
- Remember that everyone is important, but everyone cannot be number one at the same time. Know who the top priorities are, but be discreet about letting them see where they fall on the priority list.
- Negotiate realistic time lines and deliverables.
- When you cannot fulfill competing priorities, enlist the support of a supervisor as needed for additional support or resources.
- Create "tickler" or reminder files to keep track of upcoming educational events; lists of clinical references, such as the nurse managers on each clinical unit; local research colleagues; or a reminder of the steps for reports or processes that occur annually.
- Multitask as much as possible. Have extra work on hand for unexpected delays.
- Sort and prioritize tasks. If you have no deadline issues, try to complete the hardest task first.
- Identify some quiet, uninterrupted times of the day to work on regulatory writing or reading medical records. It may vary by day of the week but could be very early or late in the day or over the lunch hour when no one else is around.

Tips for Staying Sane

It is easy to get overwhelmed by the complexity and paperwork of research. Here are some ways to stay clear and focused:

- Hold onto a positive outlook and minimize the time spent with people who have too much negative energy.
- Make choices about break times during the workday. Take a walk or attend educational offerings.
- Cultivate relationships with colleagues in other disciplines. Their perspective can provide new insight into how they work, how to work more effectively with them, and how things work at the institution.
- Keep the "people" part in mind. Strive to remain polite and friendly while working through everyday challenges. The highly regulated environment of clinical research and the challenges of clinical safety for subjects can be stressful. Finding ways to acknowledge the efforts of others and expressing appreciation for their contributions makes this job a little easier.
- Accepting responsibility is not the same as taking a guilt trip. Mistakes happen, and each day has a finite number of hours. Every day offers a fresh start, and learning from mistakes is the best way to avoid making future mistakes.
- While executing the plan for any task, get into the habit of thinking about an alternate Plan B (and C) and stay open to changing course if need be.
- Take ownership of your work and do your best on every part of it. Check spelling and grammar on all documents, especially e-mails. Be proud of what you work on and look for ways to complete tasks more efficiently and more accurately.
- Share what you have learned with colleagues.

Key Take-Aways

- Research personnel are responsible for maintaining a variety of administrative duties, with each requiring distinct understandings and considerations.

- Lack of proper documentation and compliance leads to serious consequences.

- Do not let everyday activities be the excuse for distraction or delay on starting to set up your research site's administrative infrastructure.

Suggested Reading

George, M., Maxey, J., Rowlands, D., & Price, M. (2004). *The Lean Six Sigma Pocket Toolbook: A Quick Reference Guide to 100 Tools for Improving Quality and Speed.* New York: McGraw-Hill.

References

U.S. Food and Drug Administration. (2012j, April 1). CFT - Code of Federal Regulations Title 21 Chapter 1, *Subchapter D, Part 312 Investigational New Drug Application.* Retrieved from *http://www.accessdata.fda.gov/scripts/cdrh/cfdocs/cfcfr/cfrsearch.cfm?cfrpart=312.*

Chapter 3
Managing Financial Processes

Identifying and managing the financial aspects of a clinical trial is valuable regardless of whether an investigator is developing a study funded by the investigator's "own time and dime," negotiating with an industrial sponsor, or developing a budget for a research proposal to a federal agency. There are so many variables involved with budgets and payments that many investigators may just take a "best-guess" approach and deal with the consequences.

This chapter provides strategies for evaluating whether doing a study is feasible, tips on the contract process and the contract language, and examples of user-friendly research accounting tools for new investigators or finance administrators who are new to research. You will also find examples of how to gain a better understanding of site expenses and ways to leverage site resources. While there are no "one-size-fits all" approaches or processes, the real-world examples provided can help you understand the variables and customize a process for more control of research finances for your research site.

Research Roles and Financial Responsibilities

The *investigator* is responsible for finalizing the study budget with the study sponsor. Some clinical trials have multiple investigators involved, and in these cases one of them, a *principal investigator* (PI), takes primary responsibility for the overall decision-making and conduct of the trial. The PI may seek input about costs and logistics from research team members or other personnel at the institution to determine whether the trial is feasible.

The *study sponsor* usually creates the research contract, which includes a budget proposal. The sponsor may be a federal agency or private corporation, and its designated personnel are responsible for negotiating the study budget and contract with the investigators at each research site. In some cases, it is the investigator who is creating a research proposal that includes the study budget, and if the proposal is awarded (accepted), the investigator's budget is also accepted.

The investigator's institution may have *contract specialists*, personnel with legal or contract experience who are responsible for negotiating the contract with the study sponsor.

Some institutions may have department-level *administrators* who are responsible for supporting the administrative research tasks in addition to managing the business activities related to the investigators' medical practice. The research administrative or accounting activities may represent a small subset of their overall responsibilities. Centralized administrators within a large university-based system may be responsible for providing support for hundreds of federally funded and industry-sponsored clinical trials. Conversely, the investigator may not have formal administrative support, and a member of the research team, such as the research coordinator, may support the clinical and administrative tasks for the study.

Typically, *research coordinators* are responsible for supporting the day-to-day clinical trial activities, which includes the regulatory reporting processes, recruitment and study visit activities, documentation, and working with the study monitors. Research coordinators who are involved with clinical trials involving human subjects are often nurses, medical technologists, or respiratory therapists.

The Research Finance Life Cycle

This chapter introduces the fundamental concepts for the financial life cycle of a clinical trial. The life cycle for financing a research trial involves (1) evaluating the feasibility of conducting a clinical trial, (2) building or assessing a proposed budget, (3) negotiating the contract for research services, (4) tracking and reconciling revenue and site expenses, and (5) evaluating the financial outcomes.

Typically, a study sponsor contacts a potential investigator to determine whether the investigator has the interest and ability to conduct the clinical trial. This process starts with the investigator providing information about the research site resources and the sponsor providing the study protocol.

The Feasibility Process

Once a protocol is available for review, the feasibility of the study can be assessed. *Study feasibility* is not a "best guess." It is a careful assessment of the benefits and risks involved with conducting the clinical trial. During this preliminary process, the sponsor and the investigator are trying to determine whether they will formally work together on the clinical trial.

Study feasibility from an investigator's perspective asks two very different questions: "Should" the investigator do the study, and "could" the investigator do the study? The "should" aspects include weighing the ethical considerations, the level of investigator interest in the study concept, and the scientific merits of the study. The "could" aspects include the investigator's current workload and commitments, an evaluation of the site's clinical and staffing resources, and a review or comparison of "lessons learned" from similar studies and prior experience with the sponsor.

The answers to these questions can be found through the investigator's assessment of the budget and resources needed to conduct the protocol and determination of the level of risk the trial presents.

The sponsor's proposed budget should be reasonably close to the site's study expenses. A proposed site budget that is too low may indicate that the sponsor does not understand or has not done its due diligence for planning and allocating support for the site. The investigator should use caution if the sponsor's budget proposal seems excessive, as this may be a signal that the trial has significant risk involved. This risk may be related to the ability to recruit eligible subjects, a tight enrollment time line, or the complexity of the study activities for the research team and the research subjects.

> ### SITE EXAMPLE
>
> *The protocol for a study evaluating an investigational drug for patients with Alzheimer's disease may include radiologic studies of the brain at more frequent intervals than would be done for "standard-of-care" treatment. If the sponsor has not calculated the fixed costs for this additional research testing and included this figure in the budget, the proposed budget can be thousands of dollars less than the study expenses that the site will actually be responsible for.*
>
> *It is unfortunately common to see a sponsor grossly underestimate the amount of staff effort needed to perform trial activities.*

Feasibility is much more than a financial assessment. The "should" and "could" questions above should be honestly evaluated by the investigator. Once the protocol has been provided to an investigator, the sponsor usually wants to conduct its own "feasibility" process by doing a lengthy teleconference call to discuss the protocol in depth and/or send a study monitor to the investigator's site to do a site evaluation visit. This process is discussed at length in Chapter 6.

CHAPTER 3: Managing Financial Processes

Once a sponsor is satisfied that an investigator and the site are qualified to conduct the study, it will want to begin the contracting process and negotiate a study budget. At this point, the investigator may have the administrator or research staff invest the time to set up a reference binder to organize the financial documents. A list of the sections and types of documents the investigator should keep in the site file is shown in Table 3.1, which will help familiarize you with the different types of documents you will be working with.

TABLE 3.1 Financial Document Binder
Table of Contents

SECTION OPTIONS	TYPES OF DOCUMENTS
Agreements	• Copies of all confidential disclosure agreements (CDAs), clinical trial agreements (CTAs) • Principal investigator signature page for all protocol versions
Correspondence	• All communication between sponsor and investigator • All communication between investigator's institution and investigator • All communication between investigator's institution and sponsor (may be maintained in the institution's central files)
SECTION OPTIONS	TYPES OF DOCUMENTS
Budget	• Budget exhibit from the contract • Investigator's worksheets • Reference documents on test and procedure costs, such as protocol schedule of events and the investigator's prices
Reconciliation	• Investigator's workbook • All original receipts from site purchases • Documentation of sponsor payments • Itemized payment details • Investigator's institution's internal accounting systems

Depending on the investigator and how things work at that institution, these documents may be maintained by the contract specialists, the investigator's finance administrator, or the investigator, or all of them may maintain their own sets of these documents.

Study Budgets

A part, and only a part, of the overall picture for study feasibility is the study budget. A study budget is only a part of the overall considerations about whether to do a clinical trial. The budget is the "dollars-and-cents" plan. Creating or evaluating a study budget is a time for the investigator to consider exactly how to conduct the study using the specified funds. The contract will have an exhibit, or attachment, that specifically covers the clinical trial budget (see Form 3.1).

FORM 3.1 Study Budget Example

	A	B	C
1	**Site example of a Budget**		
2		Start up fee	$4,000.00
3		*(Includes IRB fee)*	
4		Screen failures	$1,650.00
5		*(Up to 6)*	
6		Stipend (per subject)	$300.00
7		**Per Subject Payments**	
8	Screening Visit		$1,650.00
9		Study Visit 1	$1,200.00
10		Study Visit 2	$550.00
11		Study Visit 3	$1,000.00
12		Study Visit 4	$550.00
13		Study Visit 5	$1,000.00
14	**Total**		***$11,900.00***

The sponsor commonly uses study milestones as performance indicators and ties payments to these milestones. The sponsor is often thinking about the data it needs and may use a Schedule of Events (SOE) like in Form 3.2, to track progress.

CHAPTER 3: Managing Financial Processes

The fundamental disconnect in this particular SOE is that many study site activities that will need to be performed to get the protocol data are either not listed on the SOE or are processes that support the listed activities. Either way, they add to the resources necessary to produce the data.

The sponsor for the study needs vital signs to be measured at the screening study visit. Measuring vital signs takes fewer than 10 minutes, but the subject needs to be scheduled for the appointment and then escorted to an examination room, and calibrated equipment needs to be used for taking the vital signs. None of these logistical details is mentioned, and new investigators will not know to factor these efforts and tasks into the budget.

Sponsors may have a limited understanding of study site operations, and investigators may overlook the time staff are spending on such activities as recruitment, regulatory support, and routine monitor contact and monitoring visits. These can lead to budget shortfalls.

FORM 3.2 Schedule of Events

	Screen	Visit 1	Visit 2	Visit 3	Visit 4	Visit 5
		D1	D8	D15	D22	D29
Window plus/minus	minus 2	0	1	1	2	2
Study visit-clinical	X	X	X	X		
Study visit-telephone					X	X
Informed consent	X					
Medical History	X					
Concomitant Medication	X					
Physical Examination	X	X		X		
Body weight	X			X		
Vital signs	X	X		X		
12 lead ECG [a]	X					
Pregnancy test	X	X				
Echocardiogram	X	X				
Randomization		X				
Study drug administration		X	X			
Study diary		X	X	X	X	X
Safety laboratory tests [b]	X	X		X		
Stool sample [c]		X	X	X		
Adverse Events		X	X	X	X	X
Key:	a) local test		b) central laboratory			
	c) site to store and batch ship to central laboratory					

It is important to clarify the sponsor's definition of a screen failure. This often means that a subject has provided informed consent and has subsequently withdrawn consent or that an exclusion criterion has surfaced, making the subject ineligible to participate. For study site staff, daily recruitment activities may involve preliminary evaluation of a patient's eligibility and communication with primary caregivers prior to contacting the patient. Regardless of whether the patient accepts or declines the opportunity to participate in the study, anywhere from 20 minutes to several hours of research staff time have been spent on that patient, and this time is not directly covered by the sponsor's budget. By realistically understanding staff efforts, the investigator can factor this time into the study budget calculations.

One option for the site is to make sure the screening payments reflect payment for the time spent on consented subjects as well as the time spent on the other patients who never advanced to the screening visit. Often times the subject screen-to-enrollment ratio is 10:1 or even 100:1.

Another option for the site is to negotiate a line item for recruitment activities that reflects research staff time spent executing the study site's recruitment plan, daily review of potential patients, and completion of the sponsor's screening logs.

The investigator may get budget details from the research coordinator, finance administrator, and lessons learned from previous studies. It is important to have a "Plan B" in the event of unexpected problems, such as cost increases or changes to study operations.

For investigators making research proposals that include budgets to federal sponsors, it may be many months before funding decisions are made. The investigator needs to factor in potential changes at the research site and consider that an approved study must be conducted with a budget that was created months earlier.

There are several common approaches to building or evaluating a budget. Investigators can take a guess, analogous, "top-down," or "bottom-up" approach to budgeting. A *guess* would be a number that sounds good but has no basis in fact. If the sponsor's budget is $8,000 per subject, the investigator may think, "Wow, this amount must be more than enough to cover costs." But without an evaluation of the protocol activities and a sound understanding of site expenses, this is a risky assumption if the protocol-related expenses actually come to $9,500 per subject. *Analogous* means basing a price on the costs related to conducting similar studies. This figure may be a place to start estimating a new budget, but costs may have changed, and hidden costs may be overlooked.

Top-down budgets focus on rolled-up, or lump-sum, costs. They are meant to cover all the activities related to a specific category or milestone visit. The risk to the investigator with this strategy is that by starting with the amount that the sponsor has proposed, the investigator may try to make the expenses fit this amount. The sponsor usually works with high-level, rolled-up numbers, such as payments for start-up expenses or per-subject payments. The sponsor is looking at its time line, enrollment targets, and available funding. It may have a limited understanding of the expenses related to conducting the clinical trial at the site level and may not be able to discern the reasons for significant variation in expenses between study sites. These reasons could be related to regional differences in salaries, test costs, and overhead.

Bottom-up budgets involve identifying all the study-related costs and then working up to determine the per-subject and total study budget. This method is the most accurate way to calculate site expenses, but this process involves time on the part of the research staff and a thorough understanding of site resources.

The Budget Workbook Tool

If the investigator is taking the "bottom-up" approach to building a study budget, one option is to create a workbook using Excel spreadsheets. The different spreadsheets created will compose one electronic workbook (file) that contains all the necessary budget information (see Form 3.3, Budget Workbook Summary). The benefit is that a template of items to consider can be created in the workbook and then customized based on the information in the study protocol; the investigator's understanding of available site resources; and site costs for labor, tests, and supplies.

FORM 3.3

Budget Workbook Summary

	A	B	C
1	Labor (12 months, estimate for 10 subjects)		
2	labor PI @ X %	$ 15,000.00	
3	labor PI @ Y %	$ 6,000.00	
4	Research Coordinator @ Z %	$ 22,000.00	
5	Estimated Labor subtotal	$ 43,000.00	
6	Per subject estimate on labor	$ 4,300.00	
7	Start Up Fee		non-refundable
8	Protocol intake	$ 1,000.00	site questionnaire, review of protocol, study feasibility
9	Site Evaluation Visit (SEV)	$ 400.00	monitor visit
10	Investigator Meeting	$ 1,000.00	PI, research coordinator
11	Regulatory Document preparation	$ 1,500.00	regulatory binder, IRB submission
12	Site set up	$ 1,000.00	planning meetings, source document set up, sponsor training for GCP & eDOC systems
13	Investigational Pharmacy	$ 500.00	start up only
14	Long term storage	$ 600.00	
15	Start Up subtotal	$ 6,000.00	
16	Ancillary		
17	Investigational Pharmacy	$ 100.00	per subject, covers storage, randomization, record keeping, dispensing
18	Tests	$ 450.00	per subject
19	Laboratory-local testing	$ 1,150.00	per subject
20	Laboratory-central lab support	$ 95.00	per subject for collection, processing, shipping
21	Ancillary subtotal	$ 1,795.00	per subject
22	Subtotal of start up	$ 6,000.00	item 14
23	Overhead	$ 1,560.00	26%
24	Total for start up	$ 7,560.00	
25	Subtotal of per subject cost	$ 6,095.00	item 5, 20
26	Overhead	$ 1,584.70	26% for this demonstration
27	Per subject cost	$ 7,679.70	
28	Pass Through Expenses		
29	Regulatory Fee for IRB process	$ 3,000.00	investigator's IRB fee
30	Stipend for subjects	$ 300.00	per subject

Tabs in the workbook each contain data and information that carry over to the Summary Page. → Summary Page / Labor Research Coordinator / Tests & Labs / Invest Pharmacy

Creating a budget workbook (see Form 3.3 and Form 3.5) first requires gathering these items for references that will be used to build the workbook:

1) **Final study protocol:** Read this entire document thoroughly. Identify the study population and consider how to make sure these subjects exist at the site. By taking a retrospective look at patients and using the protocol's inclusion and exclusion criteria as a checklist, this will help the investigator calculate a screen-failure ratio and project how long recruitment may take. Take into consideration any seasonal components to when patients are eligible. If the "subjects" in a trial are medical instruments, devices, or laboratory tests, arrange for a member of your research staff to observe in the clinical or lab areas to identify the processes and variables in the setting where the device or test is used. This information may help the investigator identify the optimal areas to work in or days of the week or even the time of day that would yield the greatest study advantage. This research forms the foundation of the recruitment plan.

> **EXAMPLE**
>
> *An investigator may say, "I admit three or four pneumonia patients to the ICU every week. I will have no trouble enrolling 10 subjects into this clinical trial." However, after carefully reviewing the protocol's exclusion criteria restricting patients with renal or hepatic dysfunction and then looking back at the patient population over the previous month, the investigator may discover that none of the patients cared for in the previous month would have qualified.*

> **TIP**
>
> *Some sponsors may provide the investigator with a study synopsis and/or draft protocol and budget while a final protocol is still pending. The investigator should understand that starting the budget workup with incomplete information will not save the site time, because a reinvestment of effort will be needed for checking for changes and recalculating with the additional or revised information.*

2) **Schedule of Events:** This chart (see Form 3.4) is a high-level time/task time line of the protocol activities and is usually a protocol attachment. See the example provided earlier in this chapter.

> **TIP**
>
> - *A SOE is a valuable multipurpose reference. One should be made if it is not in the protocol or if the investigator is writing a protocol.*
> - *Double-check the accuracy of the SOE against the protocol description. Discrepancies could be introduced during the sponsor's editing process.*
> - *What you are not going to see detailed on this form is all the other research tasks that will need to be done, such as the regulatory documentation, time spent setting up for*

continues

study visits and documenting afterward, communication with the sponsor, and monitoring visits.

- *Sponsor budgets may have a format similar to the layout of the SOE. The SOE provides important information but is not a substitute for the investigator's thorough review of the study protocol and understanding of site operations.*

3) **Chargemaster:** This is the research site's internal reference for medical test pricing. This can be a comprehensive reference, or the investigator may need to contact departmental personnel for prices and related charges.

> **EXAMPLE**
>
> *The cost of an echocardiogram will include hospital charges for the procedure, medication charges for the intravenous fluid and sedation, and possibly additional fees for contrast dye. There will also be a professional fee for the cardiologist's assessment of the scans. Study personnel can check with the echo lab and see whether it can quote the customary charge for a research test.*

4) **Reference documents:** The research site's regulatory-approval processes, ancillary departments, clinical stakeholders, and courier services. Also the research site's reference documentation on effort, previous study logistics, and SOPs.

In the Excel workbook, the first spreadsheet tab (see Form 3.4) will contain a summary of the site expenses.

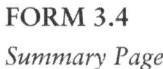

FORM 3.4

Summary Page

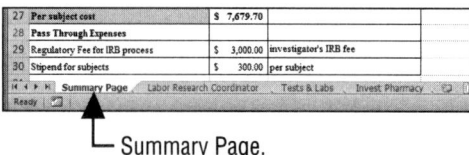

Summary Page.

CHAPTER 3: Managing Financial Processes 49

FORM 3.5 Budget Workbook *(Presented in text for ease of reading here, but should always be in an Excel workbook for calculations.)* These figures are for demonstration purposes only.

		Labor (12 months, estimate for 10 subjects)	
1	labor PI @ X % of FTE	$15,000.00	
2	labor PI @ Y % of FTE	$6,000.00	
3	Research Coordinator @ Z % of FTE	$22,000.00	
4	Estimated Labor subtotal	$43,000.00	total for items 1, 2, 3
5	Per subject estimate on labor	$4,300.00	divide by estimated 10 subjects
	Start Up Fee		non-refundable
6	Protocol intake	$1,000.00	site questionnaire, review of protocol, study feasiblity
7	Site Evaluation Visit (SEV)	$ 400.00	monitor visit
8	Investigator Meeting	$1,000.00	PI, research coordinator
9	Regulatory Document preparation	$1,500.00	regulatory binder, IRB submission
10	Site set up	$1,000.00	planning meetings, source document set up, sponsor training for GCP & eDOC systems
11	Investigational Pharmacy	$ 500.00	start up only
12	Long term storage	$ 600.00	
13	Start Up subtotal	$6,000.00	total for items 6, 7, 8, 9, 10, 11, 12
		Ancillary	
14	Investigational Pharmacy	$ 100.00	per subject, covers storage, randomization, record keeping, dispensing
15	Tests	$ 450.00	per subject
16	Laboratory-local testing	$1,150.00	per subject
17	Laboratory-central lab support	$ 95.00	per subject for collection, processing, shipping
18	Ancillary subtotal	$1,795.00	per subject cost for items 14, 15, 16, 17, 18
19	Subtotal of start up	$6,000.00	item 13
20	Overhead	$1,560.00	% will vary by sponsor and site; 26% for this demonstration
21	**Total for start up**	**$7,560.00**	
22	Subtotal of per subject cost	$6,095.00	total of items 5, 18
23	Overhead	$1,584.70	26% for this demonstration
24	Per subject cost	$7,679.70	
		Pass Through Expenses	
25	Regulatory Fee for IRB process	$3,000.00	investigator's IRB fee
26	Stipend for subjects	$ 300.00	per subject; to be invoiced to sponsor
	Summary / LaborResearchCoord / Tests&Labs / InvestigationalPharmacy		

This worksheet tells us that the startup cost is $7,560.00, that the cost per subject (labor and ancillary testing) is $6,095.00, and that the cost of other fees (IRB and stipends) is $6,000.00.

Create a template for the study summary page and modify the template for each study to ensure that items to consider will not be overlooked (see the appendix for more information about modifying the template). This page should give the investigator a summary of where the site costs are coming from and will become a reference tool for the negotiation discussions. It also serves as a reference for setting up the site's grant account reconciliation process for expenses and revenue payments.

Additional spreadsheets in the workbook will contain specific details, such as labor coordination, tests and labs, and investigational pharmacy.

FORM 3.6 Effort Log

OPTION 1: High-level assessment of effort by study.

Calendar Day	Study A	Study B	Study C
1	3	2	1
2	4	1	3.5
3	6	1	0
4	5	0	3
5	6	2	0

OPTION 2: High-level assessment of effort by type of activity.

Calendar Day	Study A		Study B		Study C	
	Regulatory	Study Act	Regulatory	Study Act	Regulatory	S
1	1	2	0	1	2	
2	3	1	0	1	0	
3	0	6	0	1	0	
4	4	1	0	0	3	
5	4	2	2	0	0	

OPTION 3: High-level assessment of effort by task frequency.

Calendar Day	Study A			Study B	Study C
	One time	Maintain	Subject		
1	1	0.5	1.5	2	1
2	3	1	0	1	3.5
3	0	6	0	1	0
4	4	1	0	0	3
5	4	2	0	2	0

Capturing Research Labor Data

Understanding research labor allows investigators to better estimate its expense. No universal "cookie-cutter" charges for research services apply across all types of trials at all types of research sites. What the investigator can do is work on building an understanding of the research labor at a specific site in terms of types and amount of effort and employee costs.

A starting point for the investigator is to gain an understanding of how much time the staff is spending on each study by creating a high-level effort-tracking log. One way to do this is to set up a simple spreadsheet with basic categories to track time spent on each study on a daily basis. See Form 3.6.

C	Education	Admin	Paid Time Off	Total	Weekly Total
	1	1		8	
				8.5	
	1			8	
				8	
				8	
					40.5

C	Education	Admin	Paid Time Off	Total	Weekly Total
Study Act					
0	1	1		8	
3.5				8.5	
0	1			8	
0				8	
0				8	
					40.5

y C	Education	Admin	Paid Time Off	Total	Weekly Total
	1	1		8	
				8.5	
	1			8	
				8	
				8	
					40.5

Form 3.6 shows three ways to track effort from the point of view of general hours spent on a study, hours by category, or hours by special task, such as specific regulatory tasks. By taking a few minutes at the end of the day to reflect on where time has been used, these important data are easily tracked. Start with several large categories, such as a column for each study, and add a few additional categories, such as education and administrative time. The goal should be to get a ballpark figure of what was performed that day and insert the hours into the spreadsheet. By the end of the week and the month, these hours will clearly indicate where effort has been spent, and over time trends will become apparent.

By periodically reviewing effort, an investigator can identify issues that require intervention or redirection of staff, highlight performance issues, or signal when or whether the time is right to take on additional work. Effort logs are also valuable tools for employees to use for self-reflection to make the most effective use of their time and to prioritize activities. This tool can get the research team thinking about opportunities to reorganize tasks, create templates, and streamline processes. Effort logs become useful reference tools for planning future studies, because they provide the investigator with accurate information about how much time routine research tasks take.

> **TIP**
>
> *Validation of the effort logs may be important, as there will be inherent bias in employees' documentation of time spent. Some validation methods could include direct observation, having a discussion of the activities associated with blocks of time on the log, and making sure that logs are regularly updated and not "populated" far after the actual date. The effort of logging time and time to validate is uncompensated time, so these activities need to be as efficient as possible.*

Investigators also need to keep effort data in context with outcomes. Research effort that does not yield outcomes means financial ruin for a study site. Outcomes are clearly identified in each research protocol. When a study is a so-called "dog" that has crippling flaws preventing it from successfully enrolling a sufficient number of subjects, the investigator is wise to accept that continued effort will not change the outcome and consider termination to reduce further waste of effort and money.

The next evolution in understanding research effort is when the investigator is ready to grow the research operation. The investigator can start to look closely at the specific types of research tasks being done or take the effort log and split the studies into general categories, such as regulatory and study activities. The investigator should consider completing this level of detail on effort logs for only a finite period of time, because the more detailed the documentation is, the more difficult it is to sustain.

Knowing what the staff is doing for the clinical trial can give the investigator a very good understanding of how many and what type of staff are needed. For example, the research nurse coordinator may spend 40% of work time doing the clinical and documentation portions of a trial, 35% processing specimens for shipping, and 25% on clerical tasks, such as copying, filing, and inventory.

Based on this breakdown, the investigator may decide to hire a research assistant for delegated support tasks and free up some of the research coordinator's time to take on the additional trials. If the investigator is looking at process improvement at the study site, this effort data can also be used to benchmark performance and as a performance appraisal tool.

Signs that effort tracking has "gone wrong" include staff members' becoming too detailed in their effort notations. Excessive detail may include noting restroom breaks, a 10-minute conversation with a colleague about another trial, or a detailed interim list of what has been done throughout the day and transitioning this information over to the effort log spreadsheet. Directing unnecessary effort in tracking and documenting irrelevant details indicates a misunderstanding of the purpose of the effort log.

Effort is usually the largest study-related expense, and the success of any research enterprise rests on all members of the team working as efficiently and effectively as possible. Remember, an employee's "cost" is that person's salary, which may include paid time off, such as vacation time or holidays, matching funds for retirement, and so forth in addition to hourly pay and benefits. Large organizations have often already identified this expense, so the investigator can check with the human resources department or calculate a rough estimate of benefits by adding 25% of the hourly wage for a total employee cost.

Another way to understand research effort is to look at a study as a series of milestones. Virtually every study has planning, start-up, study visits or data collection, and closeout phases. Depending on the study, each of these phases can include many tasks and consume variable lengths of time. For an industry-sponsored drug or device trial, the planning phase for the investigator may consist of reviewing the protocol and conducting a study-feasibility analysis.

Start-up activities include assembling the regulatory documents and obtaining the necessary approvals. The study visits or data-collection activities are usually reflected on the SOE page, so it should be apparent that if the investigator only considers these activities, a significant amount of effort is not being taken into account.

Once the study-visit activities or data collection is complete, the investigator is responsible for filing final regulatory documents, resolving all sponsor queries, and boxing and storing records for years. The investigator can take the staff's raw effort hours and group them under the different phases of the study to gain a general understanding of the amount of effort spent on planning, start-up, study activities, and closeout. If an investigator is wondering whether to add additional staff or specialty staff, staff can designate whether their time is spent on regulatory versus other study activities. Three months' worth of this data should suffice to complete such an evaluation.

Other Research Site Expenses

Such items as tests, use of examination rooms, and overhead are other important research site expenses. An understanding of these expenses can be turned into a formal research pricing reference, sometimes called a *chargemaster*. The investigator can check on pricing by communicating with the business office or department managers.

It is important to understand that some tests or procedures have multiple components, such as technical fees, related fees, and professional fees. For example, technical fees for an echocardiogram may include the hospital charges for the staff and equipment. Related fees may be charges for supplies, contrast dye, intravenous fluids, and sedation medication. A professional fee may be assessed for the cardiologist's interpretation.

The investigator should be able to identify how to get pricing information for services provided at the institution. If a central reference is not available, the investigator or research staff can assemble their own reference so they have key contacts, a glossary of billing-specific terms, and the institution's related policies and procedures easily available for the next time they need to price hospital services.

The investigator should check on the institution's policy on overhead, a fee that covers the site's indirect costs, such as utilities and depreciation on equipment. This is usually a percentage of the study payment and may vary by institution or by funding source within an institution. This amount needs to be a line item on the site's budget and is not usually a negotiable item.

The investigator is responsible for making sure that the clinical trial tests and procedures are paid for by the site's grant account and not the subject or the subject's medical insurance. Time spent tracking these expenses should be included in the study effort. If research costs are passed on to third-party payers, the institution may be guilty of Medicare or insurance fraud.

Pass-Through Expenses

Certain sponsor payments in the budget may be designated as pass-through expenses, which are to be reimbursed directly without any markup in price or application of overhead charges. An example of a pass-through expense is IRB fees. The investigator should check on the institution's policy and budget for this expense. This is not a negotiable item and is not usually subject to overhead. The sponsor may request a copy of the IRB policy on this matter for its records.

Stipend payments, or compensation for study participation, are another type of pass-through expense and are subject to federal regulation. The investigator should check on the IRB's policy and guidelines for handling stipends at the institution. From a regulatory standpoint, this compensation should not be high enough to be coercive. Stipend amounts may be provided for time spent participating in study activities or to offset the expense related to travel for study visits. Stipends may be provided as a monetary payment, gift card, or meal voucher.

Form 3.7, the Stipend Tracker, can easily be modified to indicate the form of payment used in a study.

FORM 3.7 Stipend Tracker

	A	B	C	D	E	F	G	H
1	IRB#	*Title of Clinical Trial Here*						
2			Visit	Day	Date of Visit	Payment	Payment Process Date	comment
3			Screening	Day 0	6-Feb-12	$ 25.00		
4			Visit 1	Day 1	7-Feb-12	$ 25.00		
5			Visit 2	Day 8	14-Feb-12	$ 25.00		
6			Visit 3	Day 15	21-Feb-12	$ 25.00		
7	Payment					$ 100.00	22-Feb-12	subject confirmed receipt 28FEB12
8			Telephone	Visit 4	Day 22	28-Feb-12	$ 10.00	
9			Telephone	Visit 5	Day29	6-Mar-12	$ 10.00	
10	Payment					$ 20.00	7-Mar-12	subject confirmed receipt 15MAR12
11	Total					$ 120.00		

Stipend payments should be carefully documented. The sponsor will be focused on compliance with federal laws, while the investigator will be held accountable for handling, distributing, and maintaining security of the stipend funds.

The investigator is expected to comply with the institution's and IRB's policies for finder's fees, recruitment bonuses, and accelerated recruitment incentives to avoid the appearance of financial coercion.

Sample Study Budget Workbook

Entering raw estimates into the workbook can be completed with an understanding of the type of trial and protocol activities, the site's resources and staff, and site ancillary services and test costs. For demonstration purposes, we can create an example study using sample information provided.

On the Labor Research Coordinator tab in the Budget Workbook (see Form 3.8), everyday research activities that the coordinator is going to do are divided into three categories: one time, weekly, and per subject. These hours come from the investigator's understanding of how long these processes take at the study site.

FORM 3.8 Labor Worksheet

	Activities	One Time	Study Maint.	Per Subject Hour	Notes
1					
2	Site Evaluation visit	4			monitor interview & tour
3	Feasibility w/chart review	6			read protocol, create budget, retro chart review
4	Regulatory Start Up Documents	4			regulatory binder, IRB submission
5	Investigator Meeting	16			estimated 2-day meeting w/travel (total time out of office)
6	Set up site process and documents	16			planning meetings w/ancillary stakeholders, create source docs receive and inventory supplies
7	eDoc and GCP training	20			estimated hours based on protocol
8	Regulatory support		40		amendments, request for change, annual continuing review
9	Serious Adverse Event reporting		4		estimated 1 per subject
10	Daily Screening		250		1 hour per day x 5 days x 50 weeks, screen logs to sponsor
11	Monitor Visits		40		10 hours x estimated 4 visits
12	Query Resolution		20		estimated hours based on protocol
13	Study Visits Screening - visit 9			12	estimated hours based on protocol; this per-subject number of hours needs to be multiplied by the number of subjects expected in year 1 of the study
14	Study CloseOut	12			regulatory, supply return, inventory and pack records for storage
15	Subtotal	78	354	120	
16	Total Raw Hours: 78 + 354 + 120 = 552 = 27% of a full-time employee (FTE); Multiply 27% FTE X (salary + benefits) = $27,600				

* Reminder: The numbers here are for example only and do not reflect true costs or true effort hours.

Examples of one-time activities include going to the initial investigator's meeting; preparing documents for regulatory submissions, such as initial approval or amendments; completing an annual review of the study results; and reporting serious adverse events. Weekly activities are going to include recruiting and screening for subjects, monitoring sponsor and study communication, completing and submitting screening logs, filing and planning, and updating the investigator about the study's progress. Per-subject activities refer to the study-visit activities, as described in the protocol.

It is important to remember that study visits involve more than the face-to-face time with a subject. Research personnel need to prepare for the study visit and may be doing telephone reminders, gathering supplies for specimen collection, scheduling, and entering research orders. Once the subject has left, study specimens may need to be processed and shipped, research charges for the protocol tests need to be reviewed and assigned to the correct grant account, and data may need to be pulled from the patient's medical record. Then, site research personnel need to enter data into the sponsor's online database.

On the Tests and Laboratory Tests spreadsheet in the workbook (Form 3.9) such specifics as the test type, frequency that it will be done for the protocol, and prices are noted to calculate the protocol-specific test prices. There are two main types of laboratory testing: those that are processed "locally" at the investigator's institution or those that are processed "centrally" at a laboratory designated by the sponsor.

"Local" laboratory charges usually include the collection, processing, and analysis of specimens. The investigator's institution will have a reference identifying the test cost. The investigator should make sure to understand the institution's policies on pricing and whether some or all research tests are provided at a discounted price. One simple spreadsheet design indicates the test, frequency, and cost to allow the investigator to arrive at a per-subject test cost.

"Central" laboratory test charges are paid for directly by the sponsor. However, site costs are associated with time spent preparing research samples for shipping and learning the study-specific shipping procedures. Specimen-collection and processing fees may also be charged. Research staff need to complete and maintain International Air Transport Association

(IATA) training to ship biological specimens, or the investigator needs to pay the institution's laboratory staff to perform this task. It takes time to package the specimens for shipment and contact the courier to pick up or drop off the shipment. Holding specimens in a freezer may require that the investigator maintain this type of equipment, or the investigator's institution may charge a fee for using space in its freezer.

FORM 3.9 Tests and Laboratory Tests

	A	B	C	D	E	F	G	H	I	J	K
1	Example Tests & Laboratory Tests					note: demonstration purposes only; all prices are imaginary					
2				Internal Reference Number	Volume	Inpatient Technical Fee	subtotal	Research Rate	Professional Fee	Other	Per Subject total
3		Tests									
4			ECG		2	$ 300.00	$ 600.00	$ 250.00	$ 200.00		$ 450.00
5			subtotal								$ 450.00
6		Local Labs									
7			blood: chemistry panel		3	$ 395.00	$ 1,185.00	$ 425.00	$ -		$ 425.00
8			blood: hematology panel		3	$ 400.00	$ 1,200.00	$ 625.00	$ -		$ 625.00
9			Serum Pregnancy test		2	$ 235.00	$ 470.00	$ 100.00	$ -		$ 100.00
10			subtotal								$ 1,150.00
11		Central Labs									
12			Specimen collection/ processing/ storage		3	$ 100.00	$ 300.00	$ 75.00	$ -		$ 75.00
13			Dry Ice		1					$ 20.00	$ 20.00
14			subtotal								$ 95.00
15											
16			Per Subject Total								$ 1,695.00

The Tests and Laboratory Tests form is one of the tabs on the workbook.

On Form 3.10, Investigational Pharmacy Services, spreadsheet in the workbook, details are entered about charges related to the services of the investigational pharmacy, which may include study start-up and per-subject dispensing fees; see the example provided. The investigational pharmacist may also be supporting the site evaluation visit and monitoring visits as well as randomizing subjects. In addition, this person may be responsible for receiving and storing the investigational product and dispensing and compounding the investigational product.

Now with all this information available, the details from each spreadsheet page can be summarized as a per-subject cost, which can then be transferred to the Summary Budget Workbook spreadsheet shown earlier in this chapter.

FORM 3.10 Investigational Pharmacy Services

	A	B	C	D	E
1		Fee	Notes		
2	Start Up	$ 500.00	one time, site evaluation visit, study set up and documentation		
3					
4		Fee	Volume	Per subject total	
5	Pharmacy Storage	$ 25.00	2	$ 50.00	
6	Kit randomization and documentation	$ 40.00	2	$ 80.00	
7	Dispensing fee	$ 35.00	2	$ 70.00	
8				$ 200.00	
9	*note: demonstration purposes only - all prices are imaginary*				

The Investigational Pharmacy Services form is one of the tabs on the workbook.

> TIP
>
> - Some studies will simply be underbudgeted, so the investigator who must "break even" on covering costs needs to be willing to "walk away" from a study that does not pay for what it takes to conduct the protocol.
>
> - An investigator may have professional reasons for proceeding with a study that is underbudgeted, but this decision must be made with a full understanding of the actual costs and how these expenses will be paid.

- *Many organizations are carefully monitoring their operations and costs. Supplies intended for clinical or other research-project purposes should not be used to offset underfunded study expenses.*

- *Some study budgets will have a thin "revenue-to-expense" margin, and, especially in these cases, the investigator must closely monitor ongoing effort and expenses. Sluggish subject enrollment, rising supply costs, inefficient personnel or turnover in personnel, and unnecessary process steps can quickly transform a study from a financial asset into a liability.*

- *The investigator must work to make the study operations as efficient as possible. There is a limit to what a sponsor will pay.*

- *Some investigators create a rough estimate of the study budget to include with a study proposal. The investigator may make multiple study proposals before receiving a study award. When the investigator is notified of a study award, the submitted budget is now final and must be adhered to. The study award may have constraints regarding whether and how much of the awarded funds can be shifted between budgeted line items.*

- *An upfront cost/benefit analysis can take 4 or more hours. The cost/benefit analysis should be conducted as smoothly as possible by maintaining current reference tools, creating a template on an Excel worksheet, and maintaining an up-to-date pricing reference. With experience, the investigator can do a high-level analysis and determine whether a full workup is worth the effort.*

Leveraging Site Logistics to Overcome Budget Shortfalls

What if the feasibility analysis shows that available sponsor support or the budget will not cover the clinical trial's costs? Conducting clinical trials in the acute care environment can be daunting, as investigators and research personnel work to overcome the time-consuming and costly logistical challenges inherent in the conduct of clinical research. Running projects "on a shoestring" is nothing new for investigator-initiated projects, particularly in the current economic climate. Creative approaches, collaboration, and careful planning are critically important for the successful completion of clinical research projects. Research teams always need to be thinking of ways available resources can be fully leveraged for the benefit of a study. The following is an example of how we did it.

Recently, we conducted a trial to evaluate whether bathing with chlorhexidine gluconate (CHG) reduced health care–associated infections (HAIs) in ICU and non-ICU patients. The investigator and the research team developed a collaborative approach to conducting the trial and overcame the barrier of modest funding. This quasi-experimental study required patients in a 689-bed tertiary care hospital to be bathed with a 4% CHG solution over an 18-month period of time. The statistical analysis included comparing HAI data to CHG usage.

The study utilized CHG, a marketed antiseptic product that is commonly used for presurgical bathing and skin disinfection prior to intravascular catheter insertion. Hospitalized patients are at higher risk for HAIs because of their underlying conditions, and the treatments for their illnesses allow for micro-organisms to invade and cause disease. The direct result of these infections in the United States is approximately 100,000 deaths and costs of up to $45 billion annually. The investigator's research question about whether doing something as inexpensive and simple as bathing with a disinfectant soap could make a difference in HAI incidence and patient outcomes was of interest to hospital leadership and provided the foundation for their collaborative support for the trial.

The investigator's plan was to implement the use of the CHG product onto the clinical units according to a staggered schedule and collect data on unit census, product usage, and HAI incidence. HAIs of interest were central line–associated bloodstream infections (CLABSIs), catheter-associated urinary tract infections (CAUTIs), ventilator-associated pneumonia (VAP), *Clostridium difficile*–associated infections (CDIs), and acquisition or infection due to methicillin-resistant *Staphylococcus aureus* (MRSA) or vancomycin-resistant enterococci (VRE). CHG bathing was introduced in a staggered schedule in three large cohorts of patients and in a dose-ranging fashion (initially on Monday, Wednesday, and Friday, and then every day) to better discern the effect of CHG bathing and to exclude the impact of possible confounding factors.

As should be the case with all clinical trials, a feasibility assessment was conducted to identify the resources needed to conduct the study. Taking the traditional approach, the first task was to obtain IRB approval of the clinical trial and to secure informed consent from the patients or obtain a waiver of consent. For this study, a waiver of consent was granted by the IRB. The investigational product needed to be secure, accountable, and distributed to caregivers. To administer the CHG bath, the product was added to the water in the bath basins for patients receiving bathing assistance, or, for patients who were able to shower, it was provided to patients for their use while showering. The patients needed ongoing safety and HAI assessments. Documentation involved data collection on the number of participants, product usage, patient safety, and the incidence of HAI. The result of the feasibility assessment was that a minimum of 3.0 full-time employees (FTE) would be needed to support these clinical-trial activities.

The shortfall between the feasibility estimate and the modest funding secured to support the study caused the investigator to step back and rethink the study logistics. Successful study conduct requires an in-depth understanding of the standard practices and procedures at the institution, including an appreciation for the clinical mission, communication methods, and the stakeholders involved in the numerous departments that make up a university-based medical center. This understanding provided an important means for identifying alternate study methods.

The investigator knew that the existing hospital infrastructure was already providing support for patient bathing. Nursing policies and procedures provided guidance on the process, soap products were readily available, and clinical unit–specific bathing processes, such as bathing schedules and staff assignments, were in place.

The hospital also had processes for managing medical supplies, unit census data, and infection and safety surveillance. Secure supply cabinets were located on each clinical unit, and reports on stock and user access were readily available. The system was supported by a subcontractor working directly with outside manufacturers using a *supply chain*, a systematic process for moving products to customers and technology to manage inventory. The hospital's administrative staff collected detailed census data by clinical unit and provided monthly reports to stakeholders for use with planning and evaluating clinical services. Infection control personnel called infection preventionists (IPs) tracked HAI incidence and provided monthly internal reports to stakeholders and external reports to surveillance programs, such as the Centers for Disease Control's (CDC) National Healthcare Safety Network (NHSN). The hospital had an online safety reporting system for adverse events and possible drug reactions. Hospital policy provided guidance to staff on reporting requirements and processes.

The investigator formulated a new plan for the clinical-trial logistics. Hospital administration, medical, and nursing leadership all agreed to support the clinical trial. Nursing was already performing patient baths, and, with research staff providing education, they would use the CHG product for patient bathing. Medical-supply managers agreed to provide space for the CHG product in their supply cabinets, thereby providing product security and reported usage to research personnel so that a measure of compliance for patient bathing could be documented. They worked with the product manufacturer to receive regular shipments of the CHG product and kept their supply cabinets stocked. The medical-supply manager indicated that he was not aware of anyone using the Pyxisâ (Pyxis Corporation) system for a research application, so this was a novel way to maintain investigational product security and accountability. The census data, HAI data, and safety reports were already being generated, so adding the research team to their report recipients created minimal additional work.

Under the oversight of the investigator, the specific tasks to be performed by the research personnel were education and data management. The research nurse developed and implemented an educational program for the clinical staff. The IRB approved educational materials, including patient bathing instructions for staff as well as bilingual informational sheets for patients. The research nurse presented information about the trial at clinical staff meetings and nursing practice committees, usage reminder cards were placed on bathroom mirrors and the supply cabinets, and face-to-face conversations with clinical staff were conducted to identify barriers to participation and to facilitate overall communication.

The research assistant built a customized Access database, retrieved and entered the product-usage data from the supply cabinets, and entered the report data from the monthly census. Unit-specific usage graphs were formulated and sent to the units monthly to encourage compliance. Staff were reminded to use the hospital safety reporting system, and 24/7 contact information for the research personnel was provided on the units and on all correspondence. The hospital IP provided report data directly to the biostatistician.

This collaborative trial provided some learning opportunities for the research team. Despite implementing an intense educational program at the study's start-up, there was a clear need for ongoing reinforcement of the study's purpose and the role of the clinical staff. The physical presence of the research staff on the clinical units, by doing rounds or while they were performing activities for other clinical trials, was an effective way to provide feedback on progress and to encourage study participation. During these rounds, research staff noticed accumulation of partially used product in the patient bathrooms. Through discussions with the clinical staff about this observation, the research team learned that the 4-ounce bottle of the liquid investigational product was more than most people needed when showering. Nurses, generally thrifty by nature, would "save" the remainder for use the next day and not pull a new bottle from the supply cabinet. Research personnel advised staff to have the patient liberally apply the product, using the entire 4-ounce bottle with each bath or shower and not saving the leftover product. In addition, staff were reminded that there was no cost to the patient for the investigational product.

Regularly communicating with hospital leadership, using the centralized clinical manager e-mail system, and posting results in a shared electronic folder helped keep product usage "top of mind" on the busy clinical units.

Although the trial methods were highly efficient in making use of existing systems, the accuracy of the compliance measurements was not validated. Without direct observations of clinical practice, such as the removal of the CHG bottles from the supply cabinet and the patient bathing procedures, the system may have overestimated or underestimated true compliance.

The trial results found average usage at a level of 60% for all units and 90% for adult critical care areas. The CHG bathing was well tolerated, and its use was associated with a significant decrease in CDIs in hospitalized patients. From a study perspective, the reduction in an estimated 3.0 FTE needed to conduct the study to an actual 0.5% FTE average was a "win" for judicious use of very limited research funding.

The end of the story at the clinical site is that, based on this clinical trial and data from studies at other sites, the hospital has adopted permanent use of CHG for patient bathing. To disseminate the findings, the results were presented at national conferences (Rupp et al., 2011; Cavalieri et al., 2012) and published in the peer-reviewed literature (Rupp et al., 2012).

The Contract Process

A *contract* is an agreement between two parties. Two commonly used contract types are a *confidential disclosure agreement* (CDA) and a *clinical trial agreement* (CTA).

A CDA establishes the terms and conditions for release of the sponsor's confidential study protocol, as this contains proprietary information. Once the sponsor has released the protocol and the sponsor and investigator have decided they will work together on the clinical trial, a CTA between the sponsor and the investigator or the investigator's institution is negotiated. A CTA is the formal contract for research services.

For a research project, the parties may be the investigator or the investigator's institution and the study sponsor, such as a federal entity or a company developing a drug or device. The study sponsor may delegate some study-related activities to a *contract research organization* (CRO). These organizations offer specialized services for a variety of clinical-trial activities, including contract negotiation, study start-up and monitoring, and the site's payment process. In these cases, the investigator is working with representatives from the sponsor as well as the CRO. The investigator's institution may be responsible for contract approval. In these cases, the investigator may use the services of *contract specialists* to support the negotiation process, as contract law varies by jurisdiction.

Institutions may have *master agreements*, or contract templates, with specific sponsors in place in which key parts of or all the contract language has been established. This template agreement becomes a starting point for future contracts and can streamline the negotiation process. Some of the study-specific language included in a research contract defines the scope of the agreement; the potential number of subjects the site may enroll; maximum potential payment for services; study termination language; *indemnification*, which clarifies a release from future legal action; and *intellectual property* rights, which clarify the ownership of novel ideas, tools, and publishing rights.

A *study budget*, an itemized listing of payment for specific research services, is usually included as an *exhibit*, or attachment to the contract. The budget is essentially a written offer of what a sponsor will pay for the investigator's research services.

The investigator is responsible for understanding and complying with the terms in the final contract. The investigator is also responsible for the logistics of financial aspects of the contract. The investigator may have the services of a department administrator and institutional administrators to support the receipt and reconciliation processes for study funds.

Depending on the institution's policies, the investigator may not be directly involved in the negotiation of the contract, but the investigator should thoroughly read and understand the contract terms. Some things to consider implementing or questioning include:

- The investigator, finance administrator, contract specialist, and research coordinator may each be working with separate sponsor representatives. An option for clarifying these persons, their contact information, and their roles is to create a study-specific Key Contact List (see Chapter 2). This information is also useful for the sponsor, who may be working with dozens of study sites simultaneously.

- The contract may be "silent" regarding some important logistical details. The negotiation phase is a good time to clarify logistics, such as roles and responsibilities of the personnel responsible for the payment process as well as the payment time line and the payment "triggers."

- There is no "one-size-fits-all" answer to contract language. Both parties must understand how the contract terms will affect the clinical trial conduct and site logistics after the study gets started.

- Look for special contract terms related to items with special procedures and deadlines. For example, the study site may want to invoice the sponsor for the site's institutional review board (IRB) fees within 90 days of contract finalization. Subject *stipends*, fixed payments to defray expenses related to study participation, may need to be set up in a separate account so that any unused portion can be returned to the sponsor.

- The study payment process may be automated and rely upon the electronic transfer of funds directly into the investigator's designated account. The investigator's institution may receive and process sponsor payments using automated internal processes. To effectively manage payments and reconcile the grant accounts, the investigator can clarify and, if needed, negotiate for direct notification of payments and an itemized list of the study payment milestones that the amount represents. Without these items, it is virtually impossible for study-site personnel to reconcile the payments they receive for their clinical trials.

- Vague contract language referencing payments should be clarified. One term commonly used is "payment for clean data," which may be defined as when the study monitor has verified the source documents, when the data queries are all resolved, or when the data are locked for analysis. Reaching this point could be a matter of months, until the monitor has a visit to review the site documentation, or of years, when the data are finally locked for analysis.

- Sponsors may use a "hold-back" strategy, where a percentage of the milestone payments is held and paid out at the end of the study. This option provides the sponsor with some leverage to ensure that the investigator completes the study documentation, or it may be linked to site performance goals. The investigator needs to consider what percentage of the "hold back" he or she can afford and still meet site operation expenses. If the sponsor and investigator have experience working together, the sponsor may be more willing to negotiate the reduction or removal of this caveat.

- Getting a study started takes effort. The investigator needs to understand the activities involved in study start-up and consider proposing support for these activities or evaluating whether the sponsor-proposed start-up fees are sufficient. Items that are typically involved in study start-up include the time the investigator and designated staff spend reading the protocol, evaluating study feasibility, attending the investigator meeting, preparing and submitting regulatory documents to the sponsor and the IRB, planning site logistics, meeting with clinical stakeholders, creating study source documents, and receiving or ordering supplies. The investigator should consider making this fee nonrefundable.

- In the past decade, it was common for clinical trials to be funded with designated effort levels for site personnel. Research has become more focused on the outcomes, such as the number of subjects enrolled, so it is now common to see a "pay-for-performance" structure in which payments are tied to study milestones, such as subject enrollment or completed study visits. When sponsor payments are tied to enrollment, it becomes especially important to consider requesting a nonrefundable start-up fee.

- The sponsor may propose spreading out the milestone payments relatively evenly throughout the entire study time line, but this arrangement may not be in the investigator's best interest if the study-visit activities are "front-loaded" or occur during the first few study visits in the clinical trial. Evening out payments means that the payments do not keep pace with site expenditures, which can result in additional pressure on the investigator to maintain financial stability.

- Arranging contracts is a dialogue or a negotiation. Everything in a contract is open to discussion by both parties.

Reconciling Payments

Although it is important to understand the cost of performing a clinical trial at the research site and favorably negotiating the research contract, it is just as important to make sure that sponsor payments to the research site are appropriate and that record keeping is accurate. See Form 3.11, the Sponsor Payment-Remittance Detail example.

FORM 3.11 Sponsor Payment-Remittance Detail

Batch # xxx		Name of Research Site	
Trial Number yyyyy	Site Number:	Investigator	

Subject ID Num	Payment for	Amount Due
9-0004	Screening Visit	$1650.00
9-0004	Study Visit 1	$1200.00

Sponsor XXXXXX

Trial Number YYYYYY

Payment Remittance

Name of Person at Research Site

Research Site Address

The contract identifies the budgeted payment milestones, the responsible parties for processing the payments, and the investigator's contact information. When a payment arrives in the form of a paper check or electronic transfer, a Payment-Reconciliation Log (see Form 3.12) will help the site reconcile payments against the study milestones. See the example provided here.

Once again, a simple Excel spreadsheet will serve as a balance sheet. The person "balancing the books," be it the investigator, finance administrator, or research coordinator, can simply add columns to the study-visit log for recording the milestone study visits being paid. This system allows for an at-a-glance review of where milestone payments stand.

FORM 3.12 Payment-Reconciliation Log

	A	B	C	D	E	F	G	H	I
1	Protocol Title:								
2		Scr	Pmt from Sponsor	Visit 1	Pmt from Sponsor	Visit 2	Visit 3	Visit 4	Visit 5
3				D1		D8	D15	D22	D29
4	Window plus/minus	minus 2		0		1	1	2	2
5	Subject 9-0001								
6	Subject 9-0002								
7	Subject 9-0003								
8	Subject 9-0004	6-Feb-12	$ 1,650.00	7-Feb-12	$ 1,200.00	14-Feb-12	21-Feb-12	28-Feb-12	6-Mar-12
9	Subject 9-0005								
10	Subject 9-0006								
11	a: local test		b: central laboratory			c: site to store and batch ship to central laboratory			

A spreadsheet can be created which summarizes all subjects and expected payments.

Assessing the Financial Outcomes of a Clinical Trial

The ending of a clinical trial presents an opportunity to review its financial outcomes. This type of review can compare total revenue (money received from the study sponsor) to total expense. Beyond this obvious comparison, much can be learned from reviewing total staff hours against outcomes to see how the projected labor in the budget compared to the actual labor, which is invaluable knowledge for evaluating future clinical trials. The investigator can also review effort to tasks if changes in staffing models, such as adding a regulatory specialist or a research assistant, are being considered. See Form 3.13, Summary of a Clinical Trial, provided here for how to set up a spreadsheet to summarize a trial's finances.

FORM 3.13 Financial Workbook

	A	B	C	D	E	F	G
1	Received	Date	Amount		date here	Total Revenue	$ 24,350.00
2	Payment #1	5-Jan-12	$ 22,500.00		date here	Total Site Expense	$ 16,533.32
3	Payment #2	3-Apr-12	$ 1,850.00				
4	Total Revenue to date		$ 24,350.00				
5	Research Personnel			Labor			Total to date
6		Jan-12	Feb-12	Mar-12	Apr-12	May-12	
7	Principal Invest	$1,250.00	$ 1,250.00	$ 1,250.00	$ 1,250.00		
8	Secondary Invest	$ 500.00	$ 500.00	$ 500.00	$ 500.00		
9	Research Coord	$1,833.33	$ 1,833.33	$ 1,833.33	$ 1,833.33		
10	Total Salary to date	$3,583.33	$ 3,583.33	$ 3,583.33	$ 3,583.33		$ 14,333.32
11							
12	Site Expenses	Expense					Total to date
13		Jan-12	Feb-12	Mar-12	Apr-12	May-12	
14	ECG		$ 300.00				
15	laboratory tests		$ 1,000.00				
16	Invest Pharmacy fees	$ 500.00	$ 400.00				
17	Total Expense to date	$ 500.00	$ 1,700.00				$ 2,200.00

The spreadsheet can reflect payments, salaries, and study expenses for an at-a-glance review.

> **TIP**
>
> *A trial's conclusion is also an outstanding opportunity to make summary notes about the sponsor while the "lessons learned" about the sponsor and type of effort needed for the type of trial and unexpected challenges are still fresh.*

Creating a Resource Network

The investigator can check for internal support options to see whether a centralized research resource identifies other trials going on in the institution that he or she can refer to or establish collaborations. Every contact for a potential study can be kept for periodic assessment and planning purposes.

Networking with colleagues can help experienced investigators who are looking for secondary investigators or mid-level providers, such as nurse practitioners (NPs). New investigators interested in becoming involved in clinical trials may seek out opportunities to collaborate with their more experienced colleagues.

Many clinical trials have multidisciplinary components, and collaboration with colleagues is very practical. The investigator's plan for the research enterprise may include building a collaborative team of research professionals with expertise with statistics, clinical and ancillary specialists, and bench researchers. A seasoned investigator may have the research infrastructure with experienced staff and share these resources on a collaborative project. Individual members of this collaborative team may find funding opportunities for their projects and include the overall group on certain aspects of the project.

"Holes in the Boat": Common Ways Sites Can Lose Focus and Dollars

Research performance can be improved by understanding and managing site expenses. The business of research also involves identifying the hidden costs in operations. These are "holes in the boat" that can hold back the research, make progress more difficult than it needs to be, or even sink the research endeavor altogether. It is important for an investigator to take the time to do this, because so many facets of a trial introduce risks and challenges, both seen and unforeseen:

1) Once the investigator has obtained the regulatory approvals, start-up activities for the site have been completed, and the first several subjects have been enrolled, it will be apparent whether the budget is sufficient. If there is a small deficit, the investigator may be able to modify site operations to increase efficiency and still break even. If there is a considerable deficit, for any of a number of reasons or mistakes in planning, enrollment may cease. This situation would be a strong indication for at least discussing, and potentially renegotiating, the budget with the sponsor.

2) Sometimes a clinical trial needs to increase the number of study sites to accelerate enrollment and meet planned time lines. These

secondary sites are commonly called "add-on sites." Because many studies have competitive enrollment, the secondary sites should clarify the enrollment goals and status of enrollment, number of other participating sites, and the usual time line for securing regulatory approvals and site setup, and they should be certain they have a sufficient pool of eligible subjects. Only nimble sites should consider this course of action.

3) If an investigator is considering conducting a study that is in progress, he or she should ask the sponsor for feedback about the main reasons for prescreening and screening failures. Sponsors carefully monitor the inclusion and exclusion criteria in an effort to understand the barriers to enrollment. If most patients do not qualify because they do not want to come in for 15 study visits in 3 months or they have an underlying immune-compromised status, the potential add-on-site investigator should look very closely at the potential patient pool. As previously recommended, the investigator should exert due diligence by conducting a retrospective review of the patient population to better assess whether an adequate or eligible subject population truly exists at the institution.

4) The investigator may integrate research activities into the clinical practice. Clinical staff often do not clearly understand the difference between research and clinical responsibilities. Some investigators may not have many clinical trials open and may try to create composite clinical/research positions. The challenge of these competing priorities can often lead to clinical tasks' taking the majority of the staff time. In many instances, it will probably not be long until the coordinator with the split role "splits."

5) The collections process for research payments from sponsors may be handled by the investigator's finance administrator or the research coordinator. The challenge is that the finance administrator may have a limited understanding of research, and the research coordinator may have a limited understanding of accounting principles. One option is to develop a collaborative process where the research coordinator contributes information about the study milestones, status of the study, and subject visit dates and supports the reconciliation of ancillary and test charges to the grant account. The finance administrator can manage sponsor communication, summary reports to the investigator, and internal financial processes for payroll and grant account management.

> **EXAMPLE**
>
> *A sponsor provided a study synopsis to the investigator and insisted on scheduling and conducting the site-evaluation visit quickly, citing reasons of efficiency. The sponsor promised to bring a copy of the full protocol to the visit. At the time of the site-evaluation visit, detailed study information was provided, and the investigator realized it would not be likely that he would be able to enroll subjects. Perhaps the sponsor realized that it would be rejected based on the preliminary review of the protocol and hoped that its representative would be able to favorably present the study and overcome the challenges. Instead, from the site's perspective, 30 minutes of the investigator's time and 4 hours of the staff's time were wasted. The investigator should have understood that time spent supporting the site-evaluation visit displaced the staff's other commitments, such as recruitment activities or regulatory work on existing studies. Can the site-evaluation visit realistically be conducted in 2 or 4 hours? Without negotiating and controlling expectations, a site-evaluation visit can easily take 8 hours.*

Although it is not in the scope of the discussion in this book, investigators, after gaining some experience with some financially sound clinical trials, can begin to see the steps beyond the financial life cycle of a single clinical trial. These steps include establishing strategic working relationships with study sponsors, identifying and targeting funding sources, managing multiple clinical trial accounts, and forecasting and planning the financial course of their clinical trials.

Key Take-Aways

- The financial aspects of conducting a clinical trial are important to every research enterprise, whether the investigator has a "mom-and-pop shop" or is leading a vast and bustling research office.
- By building the financial infrastructure and carefully evaluating the feasibility of each study, investigators and their staff will be able to continue conducting productive clinical trials.

Suggested Reading

Harvey, G. (2013). *Excel 2013 for dummies.* Indianapolis: Wiley.

References

Cavalieri, R. J., Fitzgerald, T., Kucera, J., Malashock, C., Romero, I., & Tyner, K. Leveraging infrastructure for clinical trial conduct. SoCRA 2012 International Conference, Las Vegas, Nevada, September 21–23.

Rupp, M. E., Cavalieri, R. J., Lyden, E., Kucera, J., Martin, M., Fitzgerald, T., & VanSchooneveld, T. C. (2011). Hospital-wide chlorhexidine bathing project. *SHEA Abstract #503,* SHEA Annual Scientific Meeting, Dallas, Texas, April 3. Retrieved from http://shea.confex.com/shea/2011/webprogram/Paper3741.html

Rupp, M. E., Cavalieri, R. J., Lyden, E., Kucera, J., Martin, M., Fitzgerald, & T., VanSchooneveld, T. C. (2012). Effect of hospital-wide chlorhexidine patient bathing on healthcare-associated infections. *Infection Control and Hospital Epidemiology, 33*(11), 1094–1100.

Chapter 4
Managing Regulatory Activities and Documents

Regulatory activities and documents, despite or because of their complex nature, are well suited to standardization and process improvement. This chapter provides an introduction to the regulatory landscape for research with ideas and examples of how to work with regulatory boards and clinical trial sponsors. These ideas include tips for organizing and tracking regulatory-related documents and maintaining compliance.

Regulatory compliance begins with an understanding of the research professional's responsibilities. Many of the strategies presented here involve developing and then maintaining clinical trial processes at the research site, a proactive approach that helps research personnel avoid protocol deviations and maximize efficiency. The myriad details related to the reporting and tracking of research activities become compounded when the research investigator is working with multiple research subjects and compounded yet again when that investigator conducts multiple studies. Research professionals need to organize and sort single research events so they can be evaluated for relevance and subject safety in context with all the study events. The organizational tips and templates presented in this chapter are examples that can be customized into your own "mission-critical" management tools.

Research Roles and Regulatory Responsibilities

A *research subject* is a person who participates in a research trial and either receives the study intervention, such as an investigational product, or acts as a control. Prior to the start of any study activities, the subject is provided with complete education about the trial, including its purpose, activities involved, the subject's rights, and the subject's responsibilities regarding what to do and what to report during the study. Informed consent is an ongoing process that continues after a consent form is signed. Informed consent may be waived or modified for some clinical trials.

The research investigator is responsible for all aspects of clinical trial conduct, including regulatory compliance. When a trial has multiple participating investigators, a *principal investigator* (PI) will assume overall responsibility and lead the study. For more information on a research investigator's responsibilities, see the guidance document titled "Guidance for Industry Investigator Responsibilities—Protecting the Rights, Safety and Welfare of Study Subjects" (U.S. Department of Health and Human Services et al., 2009).

The study *sponsor* is a person, company, or organization that is responsible for the study's initiation, conduct, and financial support and oversees the trial activities to ensure regulatory compliance. A *monitor* is a study sponsor's representative who makes routine visits to the research site to verify protocol and regulatory compliance as well as data validity. A sponsor may delegate some of the clinical trial tasks and functions to an intermediary person or organization, a *contract research organization* (CRO), and the study monitor may actually be an employee of the CRO. A *sponsor-investigator* is a person who initiates and conducts a clinical trial.

Research coordinators and assistants work under the direction of investigators and are directly involved with subjects, data collection, preparation of regulatory documents, and maintenance of study files. A research coordinator may have medical training and licensure, such as nursing, medical technology, or respiratory therapy.

An *investigational pharmacist* (IP) receives, stores, compounds, randomizes, and dispenses the investigational medication.

Delegation of Tasks

The PI determines the research personnel who will be working on the trial and delegates tasks to them based on their qualifications. A simple spreadsheet, often called the Site Staff Task Delegation Log, can be created to track the site staff, their roles, and their assigned tasks.

A site example of delegation of study tasks would be for the PI, secondary investigator, an advanced practice RN, or a physician's assistant to perform the physical examinations and review clinical laboratory tests. The IP will randomize and dispense the investigational drug. The RN research coordinator will be administering the investigational drug. The research assistant will take the subject's vital signs and enter the data (see Form 4.1).

FORM 4.1 Site Staff Task Delegation Log

IRB#:

Study Title:

Site Name:

PI Name:

Name of site staff	Study Role	Tasks	Start	End	Initials	Site staff signature	PI signature
Mark E. Rupp, MD	Principal Investigator	1.2.3.4.5.6.7. 8.9.10,11, 12,13,14, 15,16,17,18	04AUG10		MER		
	Secondary Investigator	1,2,3,4,5, 10,11	04AUG10				
R. Jennifer Cavalieri, RN	Lead Study Coordinator	2,8,12,14, 15,16,17,18	04AUG10		RJC		
Investigational Pharmacist		6,7,9	04AUG10				
Research Assistant		16,17					
Laboratory Assistant		15					

Task Codes

1) Informed consent
2) Subject screening
3) Physical Examination
4) Evaluation of clinical laboratory testing
5) Medical history
6) Subject randomization
7) Dispense investigational product
8) Administer investigational product
9) Investigational product accountability
10) Causality for AE(s)/SAE(s)
11) SAE reporting
12) CRF/e-CRF completion and correction
13) Review /sign off CRF/eCRF
14) Query resolution
15) Oversight of lab sample collection, processing, and shipping
16) Maintain study files
17) Maintain regulatory files
18) Study budget
19) Other _____

Clinical Trial Documents

The key documents in a clinical trial to be familiar with include the following:

- A *research protocol* describes the purpose, design, methods, and plan for analysis of the clinical trial data. See Chapter 1 for more details on the research protocol.

- The *investigator brochure* (IB) contains relevant scientific information about the investigational product. The study sponsor is responsible for developing and regularly updating this information. This document includes a detailed description of the physical, chemical, and pharmaceutical properties of the investigational product; the results of previous studies involving animals and humans; pharmacokinetics and metabolic effects; safety and efficacy findings to date; and marketing activities to date.

- *Source data* are all the information related to the clinical findings, observations, or clinical trial activities. Source documents are original documents or records that contain data. They may include hospital or clinic records, laboratory reports, pharmacy records, radiology films, other reports, or even a scrap of paper that has a patient's blood pressure written on it at the time of study drug infusion.

- A *case report form* (CRF) is a printed or electronic document used by research personnel to record the clinical trial data.

- The reports from *Data Safety and Monitoring Committees or Boards* (DSMBs) may be organized by the sponsor to provide independent patient safety monitoring by unblinded experts. This monitoring is carried out while the clinical trial is active, with members of the group conducting regular reviews of the study data. An official report is written addressing safety, efficacy, and the risk-to-benefit ratios of the trial. This group has the authority to halt or terminate studies based on safety, efficacy, risk, or cases of overwhelming benefit or futility. These reports are official study documents that are maintained in the study regulatory file at the research site and are submitted to the investigator's Institutional Review Board (IRB).

Regulatory Oversight for Research Activities

Regulatory oversight encompasses all aspects of clinical trials and begins with the investigator and research team operations. From a regulatory standpoint, the investigator's responsibilities include ensuring subject safety and regulatory compliance. The investigator's organization may have specific research-compliance policies and authority over agreements and operations. The research site's manual of standard operating procedures (SOPs) should clearly describe the leadership team, chain of command, reporting structure, and the process for declaring any conflict of interest (COI).

The type of trial, where it is being conducted, and the study sponsor all factor into determining the specific regulatory bodies that are involved with the study. If activities will be performed in a research laboratory, the investigator's institution may require a protocol review and approval by the laboratory (biomedical) safety committee. If human subjects will be involved in the study, an IRB or ethics committee (EC), either local or central, will require protocol review and approval. An *IRB or EC* reviews the investigator's detailed information about a clinical trial involving human subjects prior the start of a clinical trial, when changes to the protocol are requested, and at the time of annual review. See Chapter 5 for a detailed understanding of working with an IRB.

Additional oversight may be involved, depending on the type of trial or funding source.

> **TIP**
>
> - *The investigator and all members of the research team are responsible for understanding and complying with the institution's research policies.*
>
> - *The investigator may meet regularly with key members of the research team and conduct focused reviews of the status of regulatory, enrollment, operations, financial, and sponsor activities.*
>
> - *The investigator is the first person research staff notify when adverse events or study violations occur.*
>
> - *Research staff may draft reporting documents for the IRB or sponsors about serious adverse events. The investigator is responsible for reviewing, editing, and approving this documentation.*
>
> - *Regulatory guidance is derived from multiple sources, such as the IRB, study sponsor, Food and Drug Administration (FDA), or Good Clinical Practice (GCP) guidelines. A general rule of thumb is to default to the most stringent regulatory recommendations. For example, a serious adverse event may not meet the local IRB reporting criteria but may still need to be reported to the sponsor.*

Research professionals who work with human subjects are responsible for understanding and complying with regulatory guidelines for GCP, instructions from the International Conference on Harmonisation (ICH), and the U.S. Department of Health and Human Services (DHHS) or the U.S Food and Drug Administration (FDA) Regulations for the Protection of Human Subjects Code of Federal Regulations (CFR) (U.S. Government Printing Office, n.d.).

The ICH was formed to develop unified standards for clinical trials so clinical data could be accepted by regulatory authorities for worldwide members. GCP is a set of international, ethical, and scientific quality standards for designing, conducting, recording, and reporting trials involving human subjects.

> **TIP**
>
> - *The ICH website, www.ich.org, is organized into four main categories: Q for quality guidelines, S for safety guidelines, E for efficacy guidelines, and M for multidisciplinary guidelines.*
>
> - *The efficacy section is the source for guidelines related to GCP. Research personnel are strongly advised to familiarize themselves with this information. These principles are woven into study documents and activities. The research site's SOPs should reflect adherence to GCP.*
>
> - *The ICH guidelines are instructions for professional and ethical decision-making. They exist so that investigators and sponsors can create customized site processes.*

The Health Insurance Portability and Accountability Act of 1996 (HIPAA) (U.S. Department of Health and Human Services, n.d.(a)), also referred to as the Privacy Rule, was enacted by the DHHS. Compliance was required as of April 1, 2003 and defines the circumstances for the disclosure of health information, referred to as protected health information (PHI).

> **TIP**
>
> - *Investigators can clarify their IRBs' policies for HIPAA statements in consent documents. Some IRBs will include this language in the body of the consent, while others may use a separate HIPAA form for the informed-consent process.*
>
> - *Many investigators and their staff are also health care professionals, and they should clearly understand the distinction between their roles as health care providers and their roles as research professionals.*
>
> - *Research personnel need to exercise their professional judgment when accessing records that contain individually identifiable PHI.*

The Office for Human Research Protections (OHRP) provides clarification, education, and regulatory oversight for biomedical and social-behavioral research studies conducted or supported by the DHHS (U.S. Department of Health and Human Services, n.d.(b)).

Institutions that conduct federally funded research involving human subjects are required by OHRP to comply with the DHHS regulations for the protection of human subjects. They issue a *federal-wide assurance* (FWA) that documents this compliance (Oregon Science and Health University, 2004).

> **TIP**
>
> - *One strategy for learning regulations is to keep a list of terminology and regulations in an electronic note or a reference binder. You can keep copies of the ethics training required by your institution, key IRB policies and regulatory communication, or updates, such as internal newsletters. You can steadily develop a working knowledge of regulatory relationships and rules.*

- *Research professionals love acronyms! Keep a running list of acronyms and treat them like the "new weekly spelling words" you were assigned in elementary school. Remember when you started learning a foreign language? By taking it word by word, you may find that you retain them better than when you just look them up in a glossary. Within the first 3 to 6 months in research, you will definitely become more comfortable "speaking the language."*

- *Check your IRB's website or call a member of the IRB support team for your institution's FWA information, www.hhs.gov/ohrp/assurances/assurances/filasurt.html. This core document is important to include in your study regulatory file and is often one of the first documents the study sponsor will request a copy of for its files.*

Misconduct or noncompliance by the research investigator or staff can include disregarding the regulations, committing fraud, or breaking federal or state laws during the performance of their research activities. The consequences of research misconduct, according to the 21 CFR, can include *debarment*, or exclusion from practicing research for the development of new drugs, for a period of time that depends on the seriousness of the offense (U.S. Department of Health and Human Services, 2012a). Regulatory compliance is a universal professional expectation, and misconduct can result in additional sanctions from licensing, state, and federal authorities.

Research and Clinical Laboratories

Laboratories that perform testing have different standards. Research laboratories follow *good laboratory practice* (GLP) standards. These regulations are listed in the DHHS 21 CFR 58 Good Laboratory Practice Regulations

(U.S. Department of Health and Human Services, 2012d). The investigator must comply with federal laws related to the handling of biologic materials. The investigator's institution may have a biosafety committee that plans and implements a biosafety program when investigators are working with high-risk organisms or doing research involving recombinant DNA molecules.

To ensure the health and safety of all personnel working with hazardous materials, the institution's biosafety program may have policies and procedures and an internal committee review process.

Clinical laboratories perform testing services for humans and therefore must hold certain clinical certifications, such as the College of American Pathologists (CAP) and Clinical Laboratory Improvement Amendments (CLIA) (College of American Pathologists, 2012). The Centers for Medicare and Medicaid Services (CMS) regulate all laboratory testing, except research, performed on humans.

Human subject research usually involves laboratory testing. Research personnel are required to comply with the clinical laboratory policies within their institution. While they may not be performing the actual test, there are policies for safe specimen collection and handling that will directly apply to a clinical research professional.

> **TIP**
>
> - *Familiarize yourself with the clinical laboratory policies and procedures for your institution. They contain such information as laboratory services, types of testing, specimen-collection instructions, and reference ranges for normal values. See Chapter 6 for specifics on proper specimen transport.*
>
> - *Identify how to access and arrange for research services, such as testing or specimen handling, within your institution. Identify the key laboratory personnel who provide the services and clarify collection, costs, and processing options.*

- *Maintaining research space, equipment, and trained staff can be a significant operating expense. One option is to identify research laboratories at your institution and explore options for a collaborative arrangement.*

- *If you plan to do your own clinical testing—for example, using pregnancy kits supplied by the study sponsor—your research site must be approved for CLIA-waived testing. Find out whether your institution's laboratory can help you get this set up.*

Organizing Regulatory Documents

Adopting a standardized and consistent approach to setting up and maintaining regulatory documents is strongly recommended. Each new study can start from a template or checklist, and the study-specific documents can be placed into the appropriate files. This system clearly identifies the location of each regulatory document, thus supporting document retrievals and audits. Standardization facilitates the use of all the files by backup or administrative study personnel as well as orientation of new personnel to the study. A systematic approach becomes critically important when the investigator is doing multiple trials or is part of a larger research organization where research personnel are working collaboratively.

When starting a clinical trial, setting up the regulatory filing system should be a top priority. The documents can be placed in a three-ring binder or a file drawer. Some types of regulatory documents are commonly used, but not every document will necessarily be needed for every study. Form 4.2 illustrates a sample Table of Contents and describes the documents that are typically located in a regulatory document binder.

FORM 4.2 Regulatory Document Binder Table of Contents

Binder Sections	Types of Documents *If documents are filed in a separate binder, make a note in this file referencing where these documents are located.*
Protocol	• Copies of all IRB-approved protocols • Original (principal investigator) signed signature page for protocols
Site logs	• Site staff task-delegation log • Master subject log • Site-visit log: signed list of all personnel making site visits • Site-training log: documentation of study training, investigator-meeting attendance, use of electronic documentation systems, site initiation
1572	• Copy of all signed versions
Financial disclosure forms (FDFs)	• Copy of all signed versions for investigator and study personnel
Investigational pharmacy	• Investigator brochures (all versions) • Decoding procedures for blinded clinical trials • Package inserts (if study drug is FDA-approved) • Documentation of storage location for the investigational product • Drug accountability records (if study is blinded, the IP may hold these records) • Shipping records for investigational products • Temperature logs for equipment where investigational product is stored • Shipping documentation to validate cold chain
Laboratory	• Local and/or central laboratory accreditation documents (CAP, CLIA) for all laboratories listed on the 1572 • Documentation on the status of any research laboratory's GLP compliance (a statement from the PI or laboratory scientist documenting the location, types of laboratory activities, and compliance with institutional guidelines and committees) • Reference ranges for clinical laboratory tests • Documentation of the storage location for the research specimen(s) • Temperature logs for equipment where investigational product is stored • Shipping documentation to include staff training, shipping airbills, temperature logs, and validation of cold chain
Institutional Review Board (IRB)/Ethics Committee (EC)	• IRB FWA number or list of IRB members • File copy of all IRB/institution-required ethics training done by PI and the research team • Regulatory document tracker spreadsheet • Copies of all correspondence and documents submitted to the IRB • IRB approval letters • All versions of IRB consents • IRB-approved recruitment materials, subject diaries, and any other documents given to subjects

CHAPTER 4: Managing Regulatory Activities and Documents | 89

Binder Sections	Types of Documents
Serious adverse events (SAEs)	• Master copy of the IRB SAE documentation form • IRB instructions related to completion of SAE forms • Master copy of the sponsor's SAE form • Sponsor instructions related to completion of SAE form • Copies of all study SAEs and communication between the IRB and sponsor related to the reporting of the SAEs • Site personnel may choose to also file the documentation in the subject's source document binder • Site personnel may choose to make an SAE tracking form
Study protocol violations	• Master copy of the IRB protocol-violation documentation form • IRB instructions related to completion of IRB protocol-violation form • Master copy of the sponsor's protocol-violation form • Sponsor instructions related to completion of protocol-violation form • Copies of all protocol violations and communication between the IRB and sponsor related to the reporting of the SAEs • Site personnel may choose to also file the documentation in the subject's source document binder • Site personnel may choose to make a protocol-violation tracking form
Curriculum vitae/licenses	• File copy of CV for all site personnel, with the form dated and signed in top right-hand corner (sponsor may request annual updates to these documents) • File copy of medical, nursing, and pharmacy licenses for all site personnel for the entire study period
Data safety monitoring board (DSMB)	• Documentation of the safety monitoring plan, DSMB charter • File copy of all safety-committee reports • File copy of all sponsor and IRB communication related to safety-committee reports
Data	• Templates of documentation forms • Original source documents • Description of data security measures to include privacy, security, and ethical access
Supplies and equipment	• Equipment- and supply-purchasing records for clinical trial items • Shipping records, including packing slips and items received by the research site • Equipment inventory, calibration records • Temperature logs for equipment and storage rooms
Communication	• All communication between the sponsor and study site, including electronic correspondence, facsimiles, newsletters, and notes to file (NTF) • All monitor visit letters and monitoring reports • All research site communication between site research personnel, including meeting agendas and summaries, electronic correspondence, facsimiles, and NTF

If the binder cannot reasonably contain all the documentation in a particular section, such as IRB correspondence, make a note to file (NTF) and identify the location of these documents (in another dedicated binder or file). The site may choose to set up electronic regulatory files as well.

> **TIP**
>
> *Preparing regulatory documents and managing the research site's regulatory files involve research effort. This may be a "hidden" cost of doing research for the inexperienced investigator. See Chapter 3 for an in-depth discussion of research effort.*

Also, keep documents in the regulatory files orderly and filing up to date. The study sponsor will regularly monitor them to make sure such documents as licenses, CVs or résumés, and laboratory inspection and compliance certificates are current. The sponsor may request copies of the documents for its central files.

Audits and Inspections

Investigators may be audited at any time by their institutions' compliance or IRB personnel, study sponsors, or federal agencies. Formal inspections may be performed at random intervals or "for cause." Audits and inspections may be announced or unannounced and take days or weeks to complete. The usual purpose of audits and inspections is to assess for compliance and evidence of research misconduct. The PI is responsible for every aspect of the study conduct.

Keep in mind the following about audits and inspections to help you understand and navigate the process:

- Adopt a "when" not "if" mind-set regarding the possibility of an audit and be prepared. One way to prepare is to do a mock audit and walk-through of how the process would work at your site, who would be involved, and the types of issues and/or equipment that would be evaluated.

- There may or may not be prenotification of the audit. If this is an external audit, it is important for the investigator to know whom to notify within the organization, such as the compliance officer or the IRB. The study sponsor usually provides explicit instructions regarding what to do in the event of an audit, so keep this information readily available.

- Auditors will have credentials. Ask to see them before granting access to study-site records. Arrange to have the auditor work in an area removed from the study site's routine activities. Orient the auditor to the physical facilities and ensure that any questions are answered by appropriate study personnel. Provide the auditor with the documents requested and make copies of these documents. Some sponsors or the site's internal compliance personnel may want copies of the documents given to the auditor. Participate in the exit interview with the auditor and try to address any findings. Respond to any deficiencies in the audit report as soon as possible with explanations or clarifications and descriptions of the corrective action.

- Set up an internal auditing process within your research organization. Items to include can be a regulatory file checklist, a study activity and file checklist, and financial review. Such a process is useful for quality improvement (QI) initiatives. It may also be used to provide objective feedback for employee performance appraisals. Your internal audit may uncover procedural issues, interpretation issues regarding such study elements as time lines, and frank misconduct.

- Internal and external audits take time and effort. This affects how time spent on QI or mandatory audits is financially supported and when and how audits are performed.

- Some ways to avoid "audit findings" are for research personnel to know and follow the study protocol, use the correct document versions, develop systems for data collection and storage, and maintain close communication with the sponsor and site personnel.

Fraud and Misconduct

Audits and inspections are checking for evidence of research misconduct. Research misconduct refers to intentional and recklessly fraudulent activities, such as falsification, plagiarism, fabrication, and theft. Falsification involves manipulating, omitting, or altering study data. Plagiarism is taking another person's ideas or work without crediting it. Fabrication involves the creation of false data or results. Theft involves misuse or misdirection of grant funds.

Allegations or reports of misconduct start an inquiry process, and the result will be "findings" or "no findings." Investigators and research staff found guilty of research misconduct can be debarred from future research (see (U.S. Department of Health and Human Resources, n.d., d) and face civil and federal charges. Most institutions would also take action that may result in dismissal.

Why does research misconduct occur? The reasons include but are not limited to self- or site promotion, cutting corners to expedite or eliminate work, personal financial gain, or dissatisfied employees who may be working to discredit the research site. Misconduct can occur when a site lacks policies, oversight, or accounting systems. Some "red flags" include multiple financial accounts, employees who want to work unusual hours, reluctance to turn over research or financial documents, and inconsistent processes regarding study or financial records.

Keep the following in mind about fraud and misconduct:

- Unintentional human error is not fraud.
- Understand your institution's policies for research compliance and contribute feedback and best-practice ideas.
- Be prepared for an audit or inspection at all times by staying on top of the filing for the study's regulatory documents and clarifying your site processes before an auditor arrives.
- Identify the people at your site who need to know about the inspection. If your study sponsor's monitor is coming for the regular monitoring visit, the people involved would be the investigator and study coordinator. If the FDA or an International Air Transport Association (IATA) inspector is coming, your IRB, chemical safety, or research compliance officer may need to be informed. The sponsor may advise you to contact its representative when an audit is scheduled.
- After the audit, you will participate in an exit interview at which the preliminary findings will be identified. Respond to the identified deficiencies in the formal audit report as soon as possible and provide an explanation and clarification as well as the corrective actions.

Routine Study Monitoring

Sponsors routinely send clinical research associates, also known as "monitors," to the site to review site documents and activities. The role of the monitor is to facilitate communication, verify protocol compliance, and gather the data from the study site. The monitor may be a direct employee of the sponsor or work for an agency contracted by the sponsor.

A monitor is usually responsible for multiple study sites and spends a significant amount of time traveling. The monitor's time at the site is usually limited, and the person has many items to review. Sponsor requirements vary for frequency and duration of the monitoring visits, depending upon the protocol and complexity of the data being collected. The first visit will often occur shortly after the first subject is enrolled.

Preparing for the monitoring visit includes verifying that source documentation and CRF completion are up to date and signed as required. Review the status on the regulatory documentation (IRB approvals, adverse-event documentation, sponsor communications) and ensure that it is filed and ready for review. Ensure that drug-accountability documentation is complete, accurate, and current. Complete all filing prior to the visit. Make sure all tracking and screening logs are up to date.

On the day of the visit, dedicate time to make corrections and complete necessary documentation. If requested changes seem unusual or excessive, discuss them with the monitor, the PI, and/or the sponsor's project manager. Corrections may be needed for transcription errors or changed information. Corrections are indicated by placing a single line through an error, recording the correct information, dating and initialing the change, and noting a brief explanation as appropriate. Never white out, erase, or black out an error, because the obliterated item then becomes suspicious. Assist as necessary with locating, identifying, gathering, and copying study documentation.

After the monitor has departed, site personnel need to finish any remaining corrections or tasks. If a letter from the sponsor follows that asks for further corrections or information, provide it in a timely fashion. As a reminder, all correspondence from the sponsor is filed in the site's regulatory file.

Good strategies to keep in mind for monitoring visits include the following:

- Clarify visit date, time expectations, and site personnel the monitor needs to meet with (e.g., investigator, IP) and the places the monitor needs to inspect (e.g., investigational product, research specimens, storage areas). The plans for the monitoring visit need to be evaluated for conflict of time and space with the study activities and monitoring visits for other studies.

- Mark the visit on the calendar, create an agenda, and provide reminders to the research team members. Set up a study-specific Site Visit Log (see Form 4.3) to document the visit; see the following example. Having a study-specific sign-in sheet preserves confidentiality if the site is conducting studies with multiple sponsors. The sign-in sheet serves as a site reference. For example, a sponsor once queried our study site about missing monitor correspondence. Upon our investigation, we found no record of the monitor's being on site during the specified time interval, and the sponsor was in error. It is common practice for sites to require monitors to wear visitor badges and to strictly limit their access to clinical and ancillary areas. When they must go into these areas, they are accompanied by a member of the investigator's research team.

- Identify the workspace for the monitor (e.g., table and chair, Internet access, and copy machine) and orient the person to the physical facilities (e.g., local directions to the institution, emergency exits, cafeteria, restrooms).

- Ask the monitor to identify the priorities for this visit if he or she has not already done so when the visit was scheduled and have the research records ready and filing done. A monitor needs appropriate access to the research source documents and regulatory binders.

- The investigator and coordinator need to be available during the monitoring visit to answer questions, resolve queries, and provide additional information as requested. An efficient way to handle this is to set the monitor up in a workspace and check with him or her regularly to clarify any batched questions.

FORM 4.3 Site Visit Log

IRB#:

Study title:

Site name:

PI name:

Sponsor representative name (printed)	Sponsor representative name (signed)	Date of visit	Time start	Time end	Visit purpose	Site personnel (signed)
Mary Smith, CRA		07 MAY 12	0900	1700	Site evaluation visit	
Betty Jones, CRA		30 JUL 12	0830	1730	Site initiation visit	
Betty Jones, CRA		10 SEP 12	0900	1715	Site monitoring visit	

Roaming and Credentialing Activities

Working with research subjects sometimes requires research personnel to travel within the community, speak with medical caregivers in other medical institutions, cross state lines, or enter medical facilities where they are not on staff. This is often called *roaming*.

These activities are an example of what makes research activities so exciting and diverse. In these cases, licensed medical personnel must understand and comply with their institutions' policies for travel and state licensing guidelines for their professional practices, obtain approval to enter other medical facilities, or follow additional IRB requirements. The regulatory file is an appropriate place to keep this information. If a study is being conducted under an investigational new drug (IND) application, all study locations will need to be listed on FDA Form 1572.

Credentials, such as licenses, certificates, or CVs, document knowledge. The term *credentialing* refers to the process by which the qualifications of licensed faculty and personnel are documented. This is a customary practice in medical facilities. The type of information they typically verify is current licensure, professional experience, and procedure or testing competencies. The institution will want to know the purpose of the visit and have a copy of the subject's informed-consent document, the qualifications of the research staff, and specific study-related tasks. This may be a formal process, especially if the activities are expected to be ongoing, or informal, with a verbal explanation and provision of a copy of the informed consent form.

> **TIP**
>
> *The study visits for an inpatient clinical trial may include telephone follow-up or visits to monitor safety and efficacy after the subjects are discharged. Members of the clinical trial team, the investigator, secondary investigator, research nurse coordinator, and research assistant may travel to locations or communities where multiple study participants reside. At a local clinic, they may provide education for the subjects, collect specimens for research testing, or do physical examinations of the subjects. They may also meet with local physicians and provide in-depth medical information about the medical condition being studied. Arrangements for the members of the research team in these cases may include credentialing and licensing as well as the technical arrangements for specimen transport.*

Key Take-Aways

- Get familiar with and organize all regulatory documents.
- Regulatory compliance for the research professional is not optional.
- A bit of preparatory work may yield large payoffs by keeping compliance on track and preventing intentional or unintentional deviations from the research protocol.

Suggested Reading

GCP: http://www.ich.org/products/guidelines

Investigator responsibilities: http://www.fda.gov/downloads/Drugs/GuidanceCompliance-RegulatoryInformation/Guidances/UCM187772.pdf

CFR guidelines: http://www.fda.gov/oc/gcp and http://www.gpo.gov/fdsys/browse/collectionCfr.action?collectionCode=CFR

Health Insurance Portability and Accountability Act of 1996 (HIPAA): http://www.hhs.gov/ocr/privacy/

Debarment: http://www.fda.gov/ICECI/EnforcementActions/FDADebarmentList/default.htm

CFR Title 21: http://www.accessdata.fda.gov/scripts/cdrh/cfdocs/cfcfr/CFRSearch.cfm?CFRPart=56

IRBs: http://www.hhs.gov/ohrp/assurances/irb/index.html

OHRP: http://www.hhs.gov/ohrp/

FWA: http://www.ohsu.edu/xd/about/services/integrity/policies/upload/FWA-03.pdf

Informed Consent: http://www.accessdata.fda.gov/scripts/cdrh/cfdocs/cfcfr/CFRSearch.cfm?fr=50.25

GLP regulations in CFR Title 21 Good Laboratory Practice for Nonclinical Laboratory Studies: http://www.accessdata.fda.gov/scripts/cdrh/cfdocs/cfcfr/CFRSearch.cfm?CFRPart=58

CAP: http://www.cap.org/apps/cap.portal

CLIA: http://www.cms.gov/Regulations-and-Guidance/Legislation/CLIA

Guidance Sheet for IRBs, Clinical Investigators, and Sponsors FDA Inspections of Clinical Investigators: http://www.fda.gov/downloads/RegulatoryInformation/Guidances/UCM126553.pdf

References

College of American Pathologists (CAP). (2012). Retrieved from http://www.cap.org/apps/cap.portal

Centers for Medicare and Medicaid Services. (2012). *Clinical Laboratory Improvement Amendments (CLIA)*. Retrieved from http://www.cms.gov/Regulations-and-Guidance/Legislation/CLIA

International Conference on Harmonisation. (October 2012). *ICH Guidelines/work products*. Retrieved from http://www.ich.org/products/guidelines.

Oregon Science & Health University. Document Control No.: IRB-FWA-03-01. (2004). *The Federal-wide Assurance (FWA): What is it and when is it needed?* Retrieved from http://www.ohsu.edu/xd/about/services/integrity/policies/upload/FWA-03.pdf

U.S. Department of Health and Human Services/FDA/U.S. Food and Drug Administration. (2012d, April 1). *CFR - Code of Federal Regulations Title 21 PART 58 Good Laboratory Practice for Nonclinical Laboratory Studies.* Retrieved from http://www.accessdata.fda.gov/scripts/cdrh/cfdocs/cfcfr/CFRSearch.cfm?CFRPart=58

U.S. Department of Health and Human Services, U.S. Food and Drug Administration, Center for Drug Evaluation and Research, Center for Biologies Evaluation and Research, Center for Devices and Radiological Health. (October 2009). *Guidance for industry investigator responsibilities–Protecting the rights, safety, and welfare of study subjects.* Retrieved from http://www.fda.gov/downloads/Drugs/GuidanceComplianceRegulatoryInformation/Guidances/UCM187772.pdf

U.S. Department of Health and Human Services/FDA/U.S. Food and Drug Administration. (2012b, April 1). *CFR - Code of Federal Regulations Title 21 Institutional Review Boards.* Retrieved from http://www.accessdata.fda.gov/scripts/cdrh/cfdocs/cfcfr/CFRSearch.cfm?CFRPart=56

U.S. Department of Health and Human Services/FDA/U.S. Food and Drug Administration. (2012a, October 1). *FDA Debarment List (Drug Product Applications).* Retrieved from http://www.fda.gov/ICECI/EnforcementActions/FDADebarmentList/default.htm

U.S. Department of Health and Human Resources. (n.d., d). *Press announcements.* Retrieved from http://www.fda.gov/NewsEvents/Newsroom/PressAnnouncements/

U.S. Department of Health and Human Services, H.H.S.gov. (n.d., a). *The Health Insurance Portability and Accountability Act of 1996 (HIPAA) Privacy and Security Rules.* Retrieved from http://www.hhs.gov/ocr/privacy/

U.S. Department of Health and Human Services, H.H.S.gov. (n.d., c). *Office for Human Research Protections (OHRP).* Retrieved from http://www.hhs.gov/ohrp/

U.S. Government Printing Office. (n.d.) *Code of federal regulations (annual edition).* Retrieved from http://www.gpo.gov/fdsys/browse/collectionCfr.action?collectionCode=CFR

Chapter 5
Working With Institutional Review Boards (Ethics Committees)

Research professionals and their institutional review board (IRB) are partners working with the common goal of protecting human research subjects. Learning about the IRB resources and navigating its processes can be a challenge for those new to research. This chapter provides a basic explanation of IRB processes from the research professional's perspective and focuses on examples and tips for working more effectively and efficiently with this important committee.

Research Roles and Responsibilities

The *investigator* is responsible for research compliance, which includes obtaining and maintaining IRB approval for their trials. The investigator's research staff, *coordinators, assistants, or regulatory specialists,* draft documents and maintain study regulatory files for the investigator.

An *institutional review board* (IRB) is an independent board composed of representatives from a variety of scientific and professional disciplines and the community. The IRB follows the U.S. Department of Health and Human Services (DHHS) Regulations for Protection of Human Subjects 45 CFR 46 and conducts comprehensive reviews of all research protocols involving human subjects (U.S. Department of Health and Human Services, n.d., b).

Administrative IRB personnel provide logistical support for IRB processes. They may provide education and guidance for investigators and their research staff. They may also be involved in prereview of documents for the IRB in order to prevent unnecessary delays.

Get to Know Your IRB

Investigators will have multiple interactions with the IRB during the course of their study, and each of these interactions will have a process and related forms.

> **TIP**
>
> *Developing a good working relationship with your IRB is important because its decisions are critical throughout the course of a trial.*

The IRB Process

There are some standard times when IRB reviews are conducted, such as prior to the investigator's starting a clinical trial, whenever changes to the research protocol are requested, ongoing review on an annual basis, and when the study closes.

New Study Approvals

The general process for IRB approval of a new research protocol is for the investigator to provide detailed information about the clinical trial for review by members of the IRB committee.

Each IRB will have its own processes and review requirements. Some of the common review categories are a full board review, an expedited review, or protocol that may be exempt from review. Your IRB will have detailed explanations and instructions for whichever category your protocol will be assigned to.

- Full board review means the documents undergo a formal review by the entire committee.
- Expedited reviews are done for minimal-risk protocols.
- A protocol may be deemed exempt if it meets specific federal criteria.

If you are not sure what's needed for a new study, call an IRB administrator for clarification in order to avoid delays and unnecessary work.

The IRB's review process for new protocols has the potential for several outcomes. The clinical trial may receive final approval or conditional approval or be tabled. Each IRB will have its own definition of these designations. Generally speaking, *final IRB approval* means that the investigator can proceed with study activities. *Conditional approval* means that additional clarification is needed from the investigator before final approval can be given. The designation *tabled* means that substantive information is needed, and this information will be included in a second full IRB review.

In some cases, an investigator may *withdraw* an IRB application if there are irreconcilable protocol issues. The IRB may *decline to review* a protocol until sufficient information is received from the investigator.

> **TIP**
>
> - *Your IRB may require a final version of the research protocol for its review process. If the sponsor has provided a draft protocol, check with it about when the protocol will be final.*

continues

- *An investigator should have a good understanding of how long the process takes. Review your IRB's schedule for submission and review dates. It will take time to prepare the documents for the submission deadline. Once the investigator receives the IRB review notification, there may be things that need clarification. Once notified of final IRB approval, the remaining site start-up activities are accelerated. The sponsor's goal is to get the IRB approval for the research site in place as soon as possible. The investigator needs to submit thorough and complete documentation to accurately describe the protocol. This will help avoid unnecessary delays or frustration.*

- *The new investigator may not be familiar with the process or amount of time it takes to prepare the documents and get approval. The investigator can review the IRB submissions schedule and timelines and network with colleagues to get a general idea of how long things will take. Another idea is to track the effort involved with getting regulatory approval. A record of the hours spent reading all the study documents, drafting and submitting the forms, and communicating with the sponsor gives the investigator a realistic idea of the amount of effort that is needed. This information can help with effort estimates for future studies. Even a seasoned investigator may find this information to be helpful, as it can challenge assumptions, reveal shortfalls in budgeting, or identify opportunities for process improvement.*

All correspondence, electronic or printed, between the investigator and the IRB, from approval to ongoing continuing review to study closeout, must be maintained in the study site's regulatory files. Over the course of a clinical trial, study personnel typically have multiple encounters with the IRB due to submissions, approvals, changes, and renewals. One option is to maintain the printed copies in chronological order in a study-specific binder.

The process for getting IRB documents started is as follows:

1) The investigator needs to confirm which IRB he or she needs to use. The investigator's institution may require use of the local IRB. There are also commercial, free-standing IRBs also called central IRBs. FDA regulations permit both types of IRBs to review a study.

2) The next step for the investigator is to find his or her IRB's website or user manual. This website or manual contains the specific guidelines, definitions, and forms for the submission process. The key information to find includes forms, instructions, education, and the schedule for document submissions and IRB board meeting dates. Some IRBs use paper forms, and some have electronic submission processes. The detailed instructions and information can be overwhelming and confusing for those who are new to research or conduct limited or intermittent trials. Although investigators may assign the tasks of drafting and managing the regulatory documents to their research staff, they are still responsible for the submitted information and documents.

3) The third step for the investigator is to understand the institution's policy regarding the relationship between study sponsor contract process and final IRB approval. In some cases, the contract process needs to be final before regulatory approval can be obtained from the IRB. Or it may be that the IRB review processes and contract negotiation can be concurrent with final IRB approval contingent on contract approval from the sponsor or funding source.

> **TIP**
>
> - *A simple Excel spreadsheet can serve as a useful tracking tool for each IRB encounter. This tool lets the research staff monitor approval time lines, supports investigator and sponsor discussions on approval progress, and, most importantly, helps staff avoid using incorrect versions of documents, such as consent forms. A Checklist for Regulatory Documents that lists the various documents, versions, and submission dates is very helpful. See Form 5.1 for an example. This form shows exactly when these documents were approved, which consent version is the most recent, and when the updated laboratory certifications will need to be requested.*
>
> *continues*

- *Regulatory documents, such as consent forms, may undergo updates and edits over the course of the study. Research personnel can better manage these edited documents by noting the version and date in a footer on the document.*

- *Federally funded studies may require additional submissions. Check the federal contract for details about specific regulatory requirements and the location of instructions or guidance documents. It is very important that the investigator understand the institution's and the federal sponsor's requirements and instructions for budget expenditures, reports, and regulatory documents.*

The time needed to obtain the regulatory approvals must be taken into consideration within the context of the overall study time line. The investigator should check the IRB website to find out when the IRB board meetings will be held. The IRB may set deadlines for document submission that must be met before the documents can be scheduled for IRB board review. Once the IRB review is completed, the investigator is formally notified of the IRB review results.

Request for Change

Sometimes changes to the study protocol are made while the trial is going on, and these changes must be approved by the Institutional Review Board (IRB). The change may be due to many reasons, such as the need to clarify the protocol, to modify the inclusion or exclusion criteria, or to document a change in study personnel.

IRB approval for any change is necessary before it is implemented unless the change is being done to remove immediate hazards to a subject. Check with your IRB for its specific form(s) and policies for this process. Significant changes, such as protocol revisions, may require resubmission for full IRB board review. Such changes as adding or removing research personnel may have a more expedited approval process by the IRB administrators; your IRB administrators will be able to advise you.

Continuing Review

Continuing review provides the IRB with information for an annual review on the status of the study. The IRB conducts a minimum of an annual review of active research studies. For this review, the investigator can expect to provide the IRB with specific updates on enrollment status, demographic characteristics of the participants, a summary of protocol deviations and violations, Data Safety and Monitoring Board (DSMB) reports, and any publications.

> **TIP**
>
> - *The best time to prepare for continuing review is when the initial submission is made. Review the process and data that will be needed for the continuing review.*
>
> - *A simple Excel spreadsheet for collecting the data needed for the future continuing review report is helpful to use. This information has probably been provided to the sponsor, but the sponsor may not provide the site with a report. The needed information is likely in the individual subjects' files or source document binders, and each file must be pulled to get the data. These types of tracking spreadsheets are especially valuable for studies with high enrollment. See Form 5.2.*

Study Closeout

Each IRB will have guidance on the process and forms involved when a study closes. This usually involves submitting a *study closeout* report containing information similar to the annual review form summary. The report will typically include the overall enrollment and the results of the study, if known. It is important to note that enrollment may close, but a study may stay open until all the study visits for all the enrolled subjects are completed. Check with your IRB for guidance as needed.

FORM 5.1 Checklist for Regulatory Documents

Study Name: IRB Number: Investigator:
  Research Coordinator:

Submission Checklist

Item	Submission	IRB Response	Status	Note
IRB Application v 1.1 16MAY11	19-May-11	3-Jun-11	conditional approval	
IRB Application v. 1.2 17JUN11	30-Jun-11	25-Jul-11	full approval	
IRB Application v.2.0 01APR12	5-Apr-12		approval	
Request for Change				
Administrative letter regarding change in XXX	3-Jan-12	10-Jan-12	acknowledged by IRB	
RFC Amend 1 02FEB12	6-Feb-12	20-Feb-12		
Continuing Review				
CR 1.0 02APR12	5-Apr-12	30-Apr-12	approval	
Pharmacy & Therapeutics Committee (P & T)				
IRB Application v 1.0 09MAY11	9-May-11	20-Jun-11		review date is 24MAY2011

CHAPTER 5: Working With Institutional Review Boards

	Date Signed	Fax to Sponsor	Original to Sponsor	Comment
Original 1572				
PI Signed	19-Apr-11			local lab address does not match
PI Signed	25-Apr-11		19-May-11	
Affiliation Note to File	26APR11		19-May-11	tie affiliated addresses to PI
Protocol	Date Signed by PI	Fax to Sponsor	Comments	
Protocol 8888-100 version 10MAR11			Initial Submission Protocol	
Protocol 8888-100 Amendment 1 version 02FEB12			Incorporate change to inclusion criteria #5 and clarify storage of investigational product.	
Adult Consent Form	Version Date	IRB approval	Sent to Sponsor	Comments
	v. 1.0 16MAY11	conditional approval	17-Jun-11	sponsor approval 16MAY11
	v. 1.1 17JUN11	25-Jul-11		sponsor approval 28JUN11
PROXY Consent Form				
	v. 1.0 16MAY11	conditional approval	17-Jun-11	sponsor approval 16MAY11
	v. 1.1 17JUN11	25-Jul-11		sponsor approval 28JUN11
INV Brochure		To INV Pharmacist	To IRB	
Edition 3	10MAY12	9-May-11	19-May-11	
Edition 2	11AUG2010	15-Jun-12	15-Jun-12	
LAB	Expiration	Sent to Sponsor		
CLIA - Clinical Lab	19-Oct-12	5-Nov-10		
CAP	23-Jul-11	4-Jan-10		

FORM 5.2 Subject Demographic Tracker

Name of Study:

	Total	Sex		Ethnic Origin				
		male	female	Caucasian	Black, not Hispanic	Asian/ Pacific Islander	American Indian/ Native Alaskan	Other
1	2-0001	X			X			
2	2-0002	X		X				
3	2-0003		X		X			
4	2-0004		X			X		
5	2-0005	X		X				

IRB Documents

Several documents are required by an IRB through the life cycle of a study. Setting them up appropriately and keeping them organized will help any study get started on the right foot and run as smoothly as possible.

Application

The first document to understand is the IRB *application*. Your IRB may have its own name for this form, but its purpose is to summarize the essential study information for the IRB committee review. This key reference document will contain the essential information about the PI and research personnel, the investigator assurances of compliance and financial disclosures, a study abstract or high-level summary of the protocol purpose, procedures, and detailed information about the methods, procedures, protocol risks, and possible benefits.

   1) Every IRB submission is an opportunity to improve efficiency in your study, but keep in mind that completing the IRB application is a huge undertaking that requires prep work. Here are some pointers learned from experience that can help you be more successful in submitting an IRB application:

- It is always a struggle to resist the urge to open up the IRB application form and just start filling in the requested information. *First*, it's better to read all the documents the sponsor has provided, including the research protocol; all attachment documents, such as the laboratory manual; the investigator brochure; and the manual of procedures (MOP).

- Figure out your time lines. Check your IRB schedule for submission deadlines and dates of the IRB meetings for the next 6 to 8 weeks. It is useful to start with the target deadline and count backward to set goals. Check the submission deadlines for the scheduled IRB review dates.

- Identify any other related committees, such as a pharmacy or scientific review committee, from which you will need to get approval. Certain types of research involving vaccines, genetic research, or human biologic material may also have additional approval procedures. These committees and special procedures may have submission time lines.

- Review the entire IRB application form. Once you understand what information the IRB needs, you can compare this to the information that the sponsor has provided to identify anything that is missing or unclear. You can communicate with the sponsor for clarification and can get started filling out the other areas of the application document while you are waiting for the sponsor's response.

- Clarify the sequence of events for the regulatory-approval process. Each stakeholder, the IRB, the sponsor, or its regulatory authority may have separate and specific expectations.

- The IRB will want specific documents and related committee documentation for review and may not issue final IRB approval until it has complete submission information and before the study contract is finalized. The sponsor may want to review and approve the consent form before it is submitted to the IRB.

- A federal sponsor may have its own regulatory authority and require all the submission documents go through its presubmission process. These types of details may be communicated to the investigator directly or be included in the contract with the study sponsor. The bottom line is that, for this process to flow as smoothly as possible, the investigator and site staff need to understand how all the processes work.

Now you are getting closer to actually drafting the documents:

- Assemble the study references, such as the protocol, and any attachments, such as the laboratory manual, the investigator brochure (IB), sponsor's consent template, FDA Form 1572 (Statement of Investigator), and financial disclosure forms (FDFs). The protocol and IB contain information needed for the abstract, description of study-related procedures, and study risks. The laboratory manual is a good source for details about the specimens. The information on FDA Form 1572, the FDF, and the IRB application must be consistent.

- One form to create is a spreadsheet to track the medical charges for study-related tests, a Billing Tracker for Grant Charges. See Form 5.3. This Excel spreadsheet is easy to create and provides a reference and template to reconcile the individual subject's research charges. The investigator's institution may have specific billing infrastructure in place to support directing research charges to the grant account. The study spreadsheet becomes a handy reference so that all the study-related charges can be documented in the institution's process.

- Access the IRB forms necessary for the study. Consider printing a PDF version of the online document each time a writing session is ended. It may be easier to review and edit a printed form, and it serves as a backup in case document changes are not saved properly between sessions working on completing the documents.

- Once the forms are drafted, check the forms carefully, making sure that all related attachments and subcommittee documents are addressed. The investigator edits the forms as needed. This is an example of a time where due diligence really pays off.

- Once the investigator- and sponsor-approved documents are submitted to the IRB and any other required committees, final formatting and paper copies (as needed) are prepared. The study site should consider setting up the investigator's regulatory files and an electronic file for the submission documents as well as an IRB correspondence binder to hold the paper copy. The IRB submission and all subsequent communication and documents for protocol amendments and annual continuing review can be maintained in the investigator's regulatory files. This binder allows a clear documentation trail to exist for the investigator's reference and study monitoring by the sponsor and auditors, if needed.

FORM 5.3 Billing Tracker for Grant Charges *(charge examples are made up and are for illustration purposes only)*

Name of study here

Subject ID number : 2-0004

Visit	Test Name	Date of Service	Technical Fee	Professional Fee	Total	Notes
Screening	ECG	6-Feb-12	$300.00	$175.00	$475.00	
	specimen collection/ processing	6-Feb-12	$55.00		$55.00	
	pregnacy test	6-Feb-12	$100.00		$100.00	
Visit 1	pregancy test	7-Feb-12	$100.00		$100.00	
	Echocardiogram	7-Feb-12	$1,500.00	$1,800.00	$3,300.00	
	specimen collection/ processing fee	7-Feb-12	$55.00		$55.00	
Visit 2	NONE	14-Feb-12				
Visit 3	specimen collection/ processsing fee	21-Feb-12	$55.00		$55.00	
Visit 4		28-Feb-12				
	specimen collection/ processing	21-Feb-12	$55.00		$55.00	
Visit 5	NONE	6-Mar-12				
Visit 6	NONE	13-Mar-12				
Visit 7	NONE	20-Mar-12				
Visit 8	NONE	6-Apr-12				
Visit 9	NONE	6-May-12				

> **TIP**
>
> *Consider using creating a spreadsheet like the Checklist for Regulatory Documents (Form 5.1). This may not seem as important when starting a new study, but after several protocol amendments and multiple consent versions, it will become more challenging to keep track of the documents. When you compound this by multiple studies to keep track of, starting and stopping at different times, the few minutes it takes to maintain this tracker starts to look like a tremendous good return on investment. By making this form a universal tool for all the investigator's studies, it will be easy for all members of the research team to orient themselves to the current sets of documents and status of the regulatory approvals.*

Consent Forms

Consent forms are tools for the informed consent process. *Informed consent* is an ongoing process for the entire length of a research subject's study participation. The initial process where the study is explained and all the subject's questions are answered is when the consent is documented using the consent form.

Guidance for informed-consent documents can be found in 21 CFR 50.25 (U.S. Department of Health and Human Services, 2012c). Consent forms are study-, age-, and capacity-specific.

A study may have multiple types of consent forms. For example, studies involving adult subjects will use an adult consent form. Remember, the age of majority varies by state, so this may affect whether you need the proper forms for pediatric participants. A proxy consent form is used when a potential subject is incapacitated during acute illness or chronically incapacitated by such conditions as dementia. In these cases, the informed-consent process is conducted with a potential subject's legally authorized representative (LAR) using a specific type of consent form.

Some things to keep in mind about consent forms:

- Check with your IRB to see whether it requires use of a consent-form template.

- Keep a copy of each approved consent version in the site's regulatory file.

- Keep a copy of the subject's signed *original* consent form in the study files. Some research personnel keep all study-specific consent forms in one file, and others choose to keep each original signed consent form with each subject's source documents. Copies of consent forms may be sent to the patient's medical record, but with many hospitals converting to electronic medical records, this document is likely to be scanned in and then discarded in confidential waste. The investigator needs to have custody of the original signed consent.

- Keep track of the consent version that each enrolled subject has signed. Changes to the protocol or new information that may affect a subject's participation may make it necessary to reconsent subjects. One option is to note the consent version on the Master Subject Log (see Form 5.4).

FORM 5.4 Master Subject Log

Study name:

IRB#:

Sponsor-assigned Subject Number	Sponsor-assigned Subject Initials	Subject First Name	Subject Last Name	Contact Information	Phone Number	MRN	Date of Birth	Consent Type	Consent Version
20-001	ALF	Alfred L.	Friend	911 Pepper Drive Omaha, NE 68198	(xxx) 000-0000	Z9999	01JAN1900	Adult	v. 1.0 18MAY12
20-002	MAC	Mary A.	Card	346 White Road Omaha, NE 68198	(xxx) 111-1111	Z99899	02JAN1901	Proxy	v. 1.0 18MAY12

*This document is retained at the research site and serves to connect the sponsor's study identification with the participant's personal information.

- An option for supporting the consent process is to use a checklist for making notes on the discussion and activities involved. See Form 5.5, the Informed Consent Documentation Tool.

FORM 5.5 Informed Consent Documentation Tool

Date: 13 AUG 11

The process of informed consent was conducted at __2 pm__ on __13 AUG 11__ prior to the start of any study related procedures	Individuals present: patient, patient's spouse Mary Jones, Dr. Mark Rupp, Jen Cavalieri
Questions asked by the patient and answered by the research personnel:	Where are the study visits conducted? When will we know which drug dose we got?
Consent type	(adult) proxy:
Copy of form given to subject	(yes) no Reason:
Copy of Education on Subject's Rights given to subject	(yes) no Reason:
Copy of consent placed in medical record	(yes) no Reason:
Progress note in chart	(yes) no Reason:
Consent version used: Adult v1.0 16 MAY11	

Research Coordinator: _Signature_   Date: _13 Aug 11_

- The investigator is responsible for making sure that subjects understand the clinical trial. The written consent form is an important part of this process. Do not allow a potential subject to decline to read the form, as some subjects may say, "I trust you, Doc," or "I will read this later." Clarify your IRB guidelines for handling situations related to subjects who are illiterate or need translators.

- Think about how the consent process will be conducted. Some investigators may start by handing the consent form to the subject and asking the person to read it. Subjects may find the consent document overwhelming. The lengthy, copy-heavy document can be perceived as a burden and turn the patient off to the idea of study participation. One approach is to hand the patient a consent form and talk through it page by page. By making this process interactive, the investigator can assess the patient's understanding or identify any barriers to participation. Once this is done, ask the subject to read the document while the study team steps back or arranges to return later.

- Subjects need to meet the inclusion and exclusion criteria for the study. During the course of the informed-consent process, it may become apparent that they do not qualify for participation, at which point the investigator needs to diplomatically explain that study participation is no longer an option because they do not meet the study qualifications.

- Potential subjects need to understand the benefits and risks of participating in the study. Watch for signs of *therapeutic misconception*, which describes when potential subjects overestimate the benefits of participation. For some patients, research participation offers hope when they have no other options, making them desperate to enroll.

- Watch for signs that the subjects do not understand randomization. Help them understand that they cannot "choose" their study group the way they can "choose" clinical care interventions. Some patients will hint at or outright state their intentions to drop out of the study if they are not randomized to a specific arm of the study. This is another time when the investigator needs to diplomatically explain that study participation is no longer an option.

Adverse Events

An *adverse event* is any adverse experience or change that the participant experiences during the study that may or may not be related to the study. It is vital to document these events. They may not appear to be significant at the site level, but they may represent a study-related trend or risk. At each study visit, the investigator and designated research personnel should query the subject about whether any adverse events are happening and document the medically relevant details and start and stop of such an event.

> **TIP**
>
> *Your subject may report that she tripped and fell and broke her wrist, that she notices a metallic taste in her mouth 20 minutes after an infusion of the investigational drug, or that she is experiencing nasal congestion and other "cold" symptoms. These are all adverse events and should be documented. The research protocol and the study sponsor will have specific instructions for their documentation processes. The study sponsor usually wants the investigator to document all adverse events. The investigator's IRB will provide instructions, including reporting criteria for adverse events.*

Serious Adverse Event Reports

A *serious adverse event* (SAE) is any untoward medical event that results in death, is life-threatening, requires or prolongs a hospitalization, causes significant disability, results in birth defects, or potentially causes serious harm. It is deemed unexpected if it is not described in the pharmaceutical package insert or the IB. The study protocol will identify the study sponsor's reporting requirements for SAEs. The investigator's IRB will have instructions that include reporting criteria for SAEs.

> **TIP**
>
> - *The best way to prepare for reporting SAEs is before you have an SAE. Walk through the steps, make specific notes, and have forms ready to use. Setting up a study-specific reference binder containing these instructions and forms makes the process smoother and is a helpful support for backup personnel.*
>
> - *In the event of an SAE, the first thing to do is to make sure the PI is fully informed about the event. In the event of a subject's death, the sponsor will need documentation as soon as possible. The investigator and site staff need to be familiar with the institution's policy on autopsy, death summaries in the medical record, and how to request death certificates in their states.*
>
> - *A spreadsheet is very helpful for tracking site SAEs; see Form 5.6, the SAE Summary Form. It includes example data and demonstrates how the spreadsheet provides at-a-glance information on the status of each subject and each event.*

Protocol Waivers

A *waiver* is a request for modification of a specified protocol activity. Generally, the investigator will start the process by having a discussion with the sponsor. If the sponsor approves, the investigator must then obtain the IRB's approval for the waiver.

FORM 5.6 SAE Summary Form

IRB #528-10-FB   Study Name:

Subject	Event	Date of Event		Related/ Possibly Related/ Not related	IRB		Sponsor	Comments
		start	end	*per PI*	notified	response	notified	
AAA-001								
	Bilateral PE	9-Jan-12	31-Jan-12	possibly related	9-Jan-12	6-Feb-12	9-Jan-12	
	worsening pancreatic cancer	31-Jan-12		possibly related	31-Jan-12	6-Feb-12	31-Jan-12	death
BBB-003								
	Hospitalization: intractable back pain	23-Feb-12	27-Feb-12	not related	23-Feb-12	8-Mar-12	23-Feb-12	
CCC-007								
	Bilateral DVT	25-May-12	31-May-12	possibly related	25-May-12	31-May-12	25-May-12	

Depending on the request, the sponsor and IRB may approve a one-time waiver. Repeated requests for waivers may be discouraged or declined. In these cases, sponsors may need to consider revising the protocol. For example, an investigator may request a waiver for a potential subject who has a BMI of 36.2 even though the inclusion criteria state that the BMI must be 18–36. This slight difference may not seem to be clinically significant. However, the protocol may need subjects to be in this BMI range for pharmacokinetic reasons.

Protocol Deviation and Violation

Protocol deviations and violations are terms that research personnel and sponsors commonly use to describe unplanned changes to the protocol activities.

Investigators are responsible for conducting clinical trials in accordance with the protocols, and, when they sign FDA Form 1572, they have promised to notify the study sponsor before implementing any changes. The only exception would be for an investigator to immediately implement a change to protect the safety of the research subject and then report the protocol violation.

The research protocol has specific instructions for reporting noncompliance or variances from the protocol. The investigator's IRB will have guidance on reporting protocol noncompliance. Site examples of protocol noncompliance could include missed specimen collections, study visits outside proscribed protocol time lines, or visits related to investigational product administration.

> **TIP**
>
> - *Research personnel can keep a working copy of the protocol handy at all times by including it in a small notebook, the "Study File Notebook" of essential study reference documents. The current protocol, consent form, and a list of key contact people are helpful items to include in this quick reference.*
>
> - *The detailed reports for the waivers, deviations, and violations are typically filed in the regulatory binder and the subject's source document file/binder. Investigators can keep track of the essential information, such as the date and description of the event, as well as sponsor and IRB correspondence dates by using a simple Excel spreadsheet. The study sponsor and IRB have their own systems for tracking these events and do not usually provide summary reports to the site.*

IRB Policies

IRB policies are often posted on the IRB website or are located in a user manual. Each IRB will have policies and procedures based on its interpretation of the federal and international guidelines and its institutional policies. Policies are regularly reviewed and updated as needed. It is common for the document to contain a version notation of the dates of review and approval. Retired versions are filed. Research personnel are responsible for understanding and complying with their institution's IRB policies. Contact the IRB staff if you have difficulty locating this information.

> **TIP**
> - *One idea for a review of IRB policies is to use their table of contents (TOC) as a guide and list. This list can be used to identify and prioritize policies for immediate review and note additional potentially relevant policies for future use.*
> - *Connect links to the relevant institution or IRB policies to your site's standard operating procedures (SOPs).*

Building a Relationship With Your IRB

Effective and efficient interactions with your IRB start with a good understanding of its mission, processes, and communication methods. Do not overlook the importance of the "people" aspect of this department: the leadership team, administrators, and support personnel. Research personnel can use this understanding to find common ground with members of the IRB.

> **TIP**
> - *Work on getting to know the person at the other end of the telephone or e-mail. Multiple administrative staff members are likely handling the processes of routing incoming information, checking that all the relevant information is gathered, and distributing the information to the IRB committee members for the review process. They perform the essential steps to ensure that the review runs as smoothly as possible. The IRB administrators and staff may have specific roles with compliance and education or work with specific study types, such as industry-sponsored trials, oncology trials, pediatric trials, and so forth. Look for this information on the IRB website.*
>
> *continues*

- *Keep the lines of communication open.* The administrative staff are a good resource for questions about submission logistics or study concerns. They can identify resources and solutions and readily refer investigators to IRB leadership as needed.

- *Clarify how the IRB organizes and tracks studies,* because most IRBs work with hundreds of them. The investigator's study nickname or the sponsor's name is usually not enough information for reference. The IRB system may use numbering, year, or letter codes. Provide the correct IRB identification code when making telephone calls, e-mailing, or sending written correspondence.

- *Check whether the IRB has a set schedule for submissions and meetings.* If a schedule for the calendar year is available, save it electronically to the favorites tab in your web browser or print a copy for quick reference.

- *Respect the steps that are in place for the customary review process.* If every study has an "urgent" need for review, the investigator's requests will quickly lose credibility.

- *If the IRB is local, explore opportunities to get to know the IRB administrators and staff.* They may be attending or presenting educational events. Find out whether they are open to a brief "introduction" meeting, especially for investigators and staff who are new to research or to the institution. Ask whether the IRB administrators or chairs are interested in presenting at your local research events.

- *Check whether your IRB produces newsletters or hosts educational events or online tutorials.* It may be willing to hold customized educational sessions for groups or departments within your organization.

Miscellaneous Activities and Details

Your institution or IRB may require all research personnel to have current *ethics-training* certification in addition to any sponsor-required ethics or good clinical practice (GCP) training. Check your IRB website or user manual. Final IRB approval may be contingent on all members of the research team completing the ethics training. The submission process should include a check on the ethics-training status of all members of the research team to avoid holding up the IRB submission process.

Conflict-of-interest documentation, which is a declaration of any personal financial arrangements that may conflict or give the appearance of conflicting with the research activities, may be part of your research site's IRB process. The study sponsor may also require that key research personnel provide signed financial disclosure statements regarding any conflicts.

The *IRB fees* for review services may vary by IRB and depend on the type of study review. The investigator should clarify this amount as soon as possible and include this fee in the study budget. Carefully check your institution's policy to see whether this fee is exempt from overhead and budget accordingly. This fee may be negotiated with the study sponsor to be included in the nonrefundable start-up fees. The investigator should carefully check the contract for the guidelines and deadlines related to handling these types of study expenses.

ClinicalTrials.gov is an electronic registry of clinical trials for interventional drugs and devices that provides essential publicly posted information about studies.

Key Take-Aways

- The IRB is involved in almost every stage of a study from start to finish.
- A good working relationship between an investigator and the IRB is worth developing.
- A Checklist for Regulatory Documents form is a key organizational tool.

Suggested Reading

Amdur, R. & Bankert, E. (2011). Institutional review board member handbook. Massachusetts: Jones and Bartlett.

References

ClinicalTrials.gov. A service of the U.S. National Institutes of Health. (n.d.). *About Clinical Studies*. Retrieved from http://www.clinicaltrials.gov/

U.S. Department of Health and Human Services/FDA/U.S. Food and Drug Administration (2012c., April14). *CFR - Code of Federal Regulations Title 21 Sec 50.25 Elements of informed consent*. Retrieved from http://www.accessdata.fda.gov/scripts/cdrh/cfdocs/cfcfr/CFRSearch.cfm?fr=50.25

U.S. Department of Health and Human Services, H.H.S.gov. (n.d., b). *Institutional Review Boards (IRBs)*. Retrieved from http://www.hhs.gov/ohrp/assurances/irb/index.html

Chapter 6
Managing Clinical Trial Activities and Processes

Every clinical trial involves unique and common elements and logistics. So when starting up a new clinical trial, how do research personnel determine where to begin and know what to expect? Research experience brings an understanding of the general process for the start-up, conduct, and closeout of a clinical trial. Previous studies can provide a frame of reference and templates that can be modified for the new study-specific operations and processes. This chapter presents everyday tactical approaches and example templates that support clinical trial operations for those who may be new to working on clinical trials. From the first sponsor contact through study closeout, we explain, provide ideas, and offer examples of ways to approach, manage, and problem-solve common logistical challenges of conducting a clinical trial.

Research Roles and Responsibilities

The *investigator* is responsible for all aspects of the study conduct and must be qualified to assume this responsibility by virtue of education, experience, and/or licensure. For clinical trials where multiple investigators are involved, there is a *principal investigator (PI)* who assumes overall leadership of the study.

The PI is responsible for protocol compliance and any deviations from the protocol. The PI's research team may include one or more *secondary investigators*. The secondary investigators must be qualified, again by virtue of their education, experience, and/or licensure, to act on behalf of and in the temporary absence of the PI.

The clinical trial may involve *participating personnel,* such as biostatisticians, research laboratory technologists, and advanced practice nurses. They possess specialized knowledge and skills in such areas as clinical or laboratory procedures.

The PI may delegate the tasks involved with daily operations to study personnel. *Clinical research coordinators* (CRCs) may be licensed nursing or allied health professionals. *Research specialists* and *assistants* may have training or specialized skills, such as performing laboratory procedures or building databases. The PI is responsible for verifying and maintaining documentation of their credentials and competency, providing training for the protocol activities, and supervising their work. Members of the research team are responsible for reporting issues and events to the investigator in a timely manner and may provide support in the way of detailed reports, drafting documents as well as carrying out the investigator's instructions.

In acute care clinical settings, the *research coordinator* works in clinical areas and interacts with clinical nurse managers and caregivers and professionals in ancillary areas, such as the laboratory, diagnostic testing areas, and clinics. The research coordinator has regular and ongoing interaction with the research subjects and all members of the research team. In many cases, the coordinator has diverse duties and may even be involved with the institution's public-relations department and members of the general public. In community-based settings, the research coordinator works with allied health professionals in private-practice medical offices, administrative personnel at health care institutions and businesses, advertising and marketing professionals, and members of the general public.

The *investigational pharmacist* is a licensed professional who manages the logistics of receiving and dispensing the investigational products used in a clinical trial. Their responsibilities may include receiving and storing the investigational product as well as compounding, dispensing, and maintaining the drug-accountability logs.

A *study sponsor* is the source of study funding and is often, but not always, the creator of the protocol. The sponsor is not directly involved in site activities or data collection. Sponsor representatives, also called *monitors*, are responsible for evaluating protocol compliance, verifying source document data, and training the site personnel on the protocol and GCP.

Organizing Workflow

Many sources of guidance on "what to do" are available to research professionals, including the research protocol, the study sponsor, the Institutional Review Board (IRB), Good Clinical Practice (GCP) guidelines, and excellent reference publications and books. Once the "what to do" is determined, the questions about "how to do it" emerge.

One way to demonstrate the workflow within clinical trials is to separate the activities into clinical and administrative/clerical sections. In reality, these things are usually happening at the same time. On any given day, research personnel will be interacting with research subjects, completing compliance training, and pulling medical records for data. For the purposes of our discussion, we will take a look at the typical clinical workflow and then examine the administrative workflow.

Clinical Workflow

Each clinical trial will have variation with the tasks within its milestone activities. We'll explore the central clinical workflow issues that apply to most trials.

Starting Up a New Study

Typically, a study sponsor will contact a potential investigator to determine the PI's interest and ability to enroll subjects and conduct the desired clinical trial. As discussed in Chapter 3, this process starts with the investigator providing information about the research site resources (usually in the form of a questionnaire), signing a confidential disclosure agreement (CDA), and then reviewing the clinical-trial protocol provided by the sponsor.

During this preliminary process, the sponsor and the investigator are trying to determine whether they will work together on the clinical trial. The investigator will review the sponsor's site questionnaire and complete the questions about personnel qualifications, site resources, and access to potentially qualifying subjects.

> **TIP**
>
> *Sponsors want to know whether the investigator has clinical-trial experience, experience with trials related to the medical indication for the potential trial, and commitments to other clinical trials that might compete with the proposed study. Investigators can offer general responses but need to maintain confidentiality about proprietary information, such as other investigational products or inventions.*

Site Evaluation Visit Day

During a site evaluation visit, the monitor wants to determine whether the PI and the research staff are qualified, whether there are sufficient site resources to conduct the study, and whether the PI has access to the potential subjects needed for the study. This visit is the PI's opportunity to demonstrate how well-organized the site is.

Some typical questions the visiting monitor may ask may include:

1) How many subjects does the PI estimate can be enrolled at the site? The monitor will probably want to discuss how the PI arrived at this estimate.

2) What is the specific recruitment plan? The PI needs to have as much objective evidence as possible about the site's ability to enroll.

3) Are other competing studies at the site that would divert potentially eligible subjects?

During this visit, the PI may want to ask:

1) How many sites are already active (because enrollment is usually competitive)?

2) What is the study enrollment to date?

3) Are any of the active sites finding barriers to recruiting subjects?

> **TIP**
>
> *Once the monitor arrives and gets settled, provide the agenda and ask about the monitor's priorities and desired flow of activities. The monitor's time is limited, and this representative is likely heading to the airport to travel to yet another research site as soon as your visit ends.*
>
> *Also, offer the monitor a "working lunch" and eat in the research offices or a private location so you can keep talking about the site or research items on the monitor's agenda. The monitor may have allotted time for a nonworking lunch break or manage to end the visit earlier than scheduled, but this is rare.*

Ways to make the most out of site visits include:

- When contacted to schedule the visit, the research staff can ask the monitor to identify what needs to be seen and whom he or she wants to meet. Expect the request to include the laboratory, the investigational pharmacist, and the areas where study visits will be conducted.

- Offer some available dates for the site staff, PI, and investigational pharmacist to the monitor. This person is probably traveling to multiple locations and will be trying to efficiently coordinate your site's visit into his or her packed schedule.
- Create an agenda (see Form 6.1, Site Evaluation Visit) for the visit, noting the monitor's arrival time, appointments with the PI and investigational pharmacist, and time blocked out for the requested items, such as touring the clinic area or laboratory. Designate the research personnel who are responsible for escorting the monitor and answering questions.

FORM 6.1 Site Evaluation Visit

Name of study here

Date of meeting here

Purpose: Site evaluation visit

Requested items:
- Time for research questions with the lead clinical research coordinator (CRC)
- Tour of facilities
- Meeting time with investigational pharmacist: 30 minutes
- Meeting time with principal investigator: 30 minutes

Schedule:

0800–0900	Arrival, CRC will meet at xxx entrance, review of protocol logistics
0900–1000	Tour of facility (Clinic, radiology, laboratory)
1000–1100	Discussion of site logistics with research coordinator
1100–1130	Meeting with Investigational Pharmacist (protocol review, storage temp logs, etc.)
1130–1300	Continued discussion, working lunch with research coordinator
1300–1330	Meeting with principal investigator, review of protocol and investigator responsibilities
1330	Monitor to leave for airport

- Create a folder with documents for the monitor, including a Key Contacts List (see Form 2.1), the institution's laboratory certifications and normal ranges, upcoming IRB meeting dates, and the investigator's business card.

- Communicate with the managers in the ancillary departments in your institution, as a courtesy and as needed, to let them know that you will be escorting the monitor through their areas. Managers and staff in clinical departments are very used to regulatory inspections. Do not let the monitor roam the clinical area unescorted. Maintain patient privacy.

- Arrange for a meeting time and place, such as the front entrance of the institution. Give the monitor the pager or cell phone number of a site contact in case of unexpected delays. Tips about lodging and ground transportation can be offered, but remember that monitors are professional travelers.

- Upon arrival, ask the monitor to sign the Site Visit Log (see Form 6.2) and wear a visitor badge.

FORM 6.2 Site Visit Log

IRB#:						
Study title:						
Site name:						
PI name:						
Sponsor representative name (printed)	Sponsor representative name (signed)	Date of visit	Time start	Time end	Visit purpose	Site personnel (signed)
Mary Smith, CRA		07 MAY 12	0900	1700	Site evaluation visit	
Betty Jones, CRA		30 JUL 12	0830	1730	Site initiation visit	
Betty Jones, CRA		10 SEP 12	0900	1715	Site monitoring visit	

When the evaluation visit is completed, the sponsor will use the monitor's report to decide whether it will invite the investigator to participate in the study. The question for the investigator then becomes whether the clinical trial is feasible. If the study feasibility is favorable, the investigator proceeds with starting up the study. (Study feasibility, budgeting, and contracts are discussed in Chapter 3.)

Investigator Meetings

Investigator meetings (IM) are frequently held at the beginning of large, multisite clinical drug and device trials.

> **TIP**
>
> *Many IMs are held on a weekend because sponsors know that investigators are busy with their medical practices and academic responsibilities through the week.*

The purpose of the meeting is to bring together investigators and other key study personnel (research coordinators) to conduct an extensive review of the protocol and study activities, including the investigational product; laboratory procedures for specimen collection; randomization; and electronic database systems. This is a good opportunity for interaction and team building, with small group discussions between sessions and the formal training presentations. The sponsor's leadership team and the study monitors will make a special effort to meet the investigators and research coordinators, thus laying the groundwork for a positive working relationship. In addition, it is a good opportunity to network and form professional relationships with research personnel at other sites. These relations can be invaluable when protocol-related obstacles are encountered and solutions are sought. Many times, a solution or work-around at one site can be applied to another research site.

> **TIP**
>
> - *The sponsor will usually have a travel agency work with site personnel for the travel arrangements.*
>
> - *The sponsor's travel agent will contact the designated research staff, usually the PI and CRC, to make travel arrangements. This is a good time to clarify exactly which expenses will be covered for the meeting—typically, the airfare, accommodations, and ground transportation. Meals during the meeting are usually covered. Research personnel are expected to follow the sponsors' guidance regarding where to stay.*
>
> - *Research personnel who want to extend their stay for personal reasons should discuss this request with*

the sponsor's travel agent. The sponsor can only pay for event-related expense, but hotel bills can clearly distinguish the meeting time and expenses from personal time for which the traveler is responsible.

- *Research personnel should follow their institution's policy for documenting travel. This information can have repercussions when incidents or injuries occur, so site personnel should be familiar with their institution's policies for incident reporting and emergency care.*

- *Stay in touch while traveling by identifying a resource person at the research site who could assist with communication and coverage for other research activities. Leave a copy of the travel itinerary and contact information with the resource person.*

TIP

Consider bringing a double-sided copy of the protocol, IM travel information, a list of logistical questions, and a pad of paper. Alternatively, you may load electronic versions of these documents on your secure business laptop.

EXAMPLE

The sponsor may provide a binder containing the meeting documents, a copy of the protocol, and PowerPoint presentations. Ask whether the sponsor is willing to ship a copy of the binder to your site after the meeting so this large item does not have to travel home in your luggage. If the sponsor provides meeting information on a jump drive, you will need paper for taking notes.

When going on an investigational meeting, identify the documents you will need to bring and remember that business-casual attire is generally expected. Once you arrive, familiarize yourself with the conference center and the meeting-room locations.

The study sponsor may have provided such details as an agenda with meeting times with the travel information or have left an informational packet at the hotel check-in desk.

> **TIP**
>
> - *Remember that you are representing your research site. You will be interacting with the sponsor, contract research organization (CRO) personnel, and other site research investigators and their coordinators. Your behavior and dress are reflections of your professionalism.*
>
> - *Demonstrate your interest in the study topic and convey questions in a positive and constructive manner.*
>
> - *Plan to attend all the scheduled events. The study sponsor will want to maximize this opportunity for training, and you will want to maximize this opportunity to learn and ask questions.*
>
> - *Take advantage of the chance to examine displays of laboratory supplies, study drugs, or patient diaries.*

You may find it helpful to refer to an electronic or paper copy of the protocol during the presentations. Take notes and create a summary of discussion items. Note the questions raised by other research personnel and the sponsor's responses. Summarize any sidebar conversations with other meeting attendees. Share this summary of events with other site personnel, such as the IP, who may not be able to attend the meeting.

Keep all original receipts during travel, submit any allowed expenses for reimbursement as soon as practical upon returning to the office, and keep a copy of all the paperwork for your files. Sponsors usually take care of virtually all meeting expenses, so reimbursement is rarely needed.

Regulatory Start-Up

Site personnel are responsible for setting up the research site's regulatory documents and obtaining IRB approval for the study. The regulatory documents are discussed in more detail in Chapter 4, and the IRB process is covered in Chapter 5. These files and IRB approval must be in place before the study-site activities will be initiated by the sponsor.

Subject Recruitment

The first step in recruitment is to create a plan. Gather appropriate information and tools, such as the research protocol and information learned at the investigator meeting. Identify potential resources, such as members of your research team and other sources of help, including a clinical research coordinator, a research assistant who could help with incoming telephone inquiries, and a staff assistant who could help with filing. Use the information that was learned or helpful in previous recruitments. Understanding how things work in a clinical area and reusing such tools as a spreadsheet or flyer from previous research recruitments will help you think through how the recruitment will proceed.

The second step is to create a time line with discrete goals and understand the role that time plays in research. If the enrollment period is projected to last for 12 months, you will be trying to recruit at least 1 or 12 or 100 subjects per month. Eligible subjects rarely present at scheduled and comfortably staggered intervals. Although one subject per month is a rough goal, start to think about progress on a weekly scale. Many research studies have competitive recruitment, which means that if the sponsor needs 200 subjects, site enrollment is usually not capped. Efficient start-up and aggressive screening and enrollment can help a research site achieve its goals.

> **TIP**
>
> *Look closely at how soon a potentially eligible subject can be identified. Finding potential subjects late in the day or late on a Friday afternoon may lead you to be more flexible with work schedules. People may be more readily available by telephone during the early evening. They may prefer to come in to learn about the study face-to-face or have study visits on days when they are not working, such as Saturday.*

Identify the intervention triggers for recruitment by evaluating progress daily and weekly. If the number of potential subjects is lower than you expected, look carefully at which sources you expected would create those contacts. If you put IRB-approved study flyers in a clinic waiting room that hundreds of people pass through and are not getting any calls, look into the possibility that the flyers are buried under magazines or that patients are not really waiting very long in the main waiting room. You may find that patients have a longer wait in the examination room, so your flyers might attract more attention there. Investigators often overestimate recruitment referrals from colleagues. Their colleagues may be very supportive of the research, but their clinical missions or other academic commitments may not keep your study at the forefront of their plans. The investigator could create informational packets or have a research nurse available at the clinic when referring colleagues are seeing patients. This approach may also work if you need 100 volunteers to complete a study survey.

The IRB will likely require a description of the recruitment plan and activities to be documented in the application. Its members will carefully evaluate whether the recruitment activities are coercive and therefore will likely require that any materials displayed or provided to potential subjects be IRB-reviewed and -approved.

Recruitment planning requires understanding the disease being studied in the clinical trial. The investigator is responsible for educating the members of the research team. Educational tools may include explanations and articles in medical journals or textbooks. An understanding of the symptoms, typical therapy options, and the usual prognosis will help the research staff understand what to report to the investigator and also help with recruitment and retention efforts.

Research screening occurs when a potential subject is evaluated for study eligibility and when the informed-consent process takes place. The *screening ratio*, a comparison of the number of potentially eligible subjects to patients who are approached for study participation to patients who enroll in the study, is an important indicator for research sites to monitor. For example, in 1 week, 30 patients may be potentially eligible. After the initial screening, four of them appear to meet full inclusion and exclusion criteria and are invited to consider study participation. Of these four patients, one may consent and enroll in the study. The other three may decline a discussion of the study opportunity or decline to participate once they learn about the study. A *screen failure* usually refers to subjects who enroll in a study and then withdraw consent or are found to have exclusion criteria. Consider how the barriers to recruitment can be mitigated or overcome.

Investigators and research personnel meet with potential subjects during a screening visit and conduct the *informed-consent process*, which is discussed in more detail in Chapter 5.

> ### EXAMPLE
>
> *If the clinical trial involves subjects with* Clostridium difficile, *it is likely that affected patients may be experiencing moderate to severe diarrhea and fatigue. They may be reluctant to become involved in research-study activities due to their fatigue and reluctance to venture far from a restroom. You may want to acknowledge that you understand their symptoms, be honest about the time commitments, and assure them that restroom facilities are readily available. Be prepared to take a break during the informed-consent process if the patient needs to use the restroom.*

Patient Tips and Strategies

Remember the importance of body language when presenting the research information. If you are sitting with a patient in a small clinic exam room, try not to sit between the patient and the door. Ask the patient whether to leave the door open, closed, or partially closed. These actions will minimize the chance that the patient will feel trapped. Include the patient's family or friends if desired by providing them with a copy of the consent form so they can read along.

Patients may have opinions about the randomization part of the study. They may really want to be assigned to a particular cohort of the study, such as the one that gets the active research drug or the placebo cohort. Look for signs that they are only consenting until they find out which cohort they are randomized to, as they may immediately withdraw from the study if they do not get assigned to the cohort of their choice.

Research participation may be the last hope for a patient or the patient's family. Use caution during the informed-consent process and watch for signs that the patients are trying to say whatever is needed to qualify for the study. Studies about Alzheimer's disease and oncology trials are examples of clinical trials that patients may be trying hard to get into.

Carefully watch for nonverbal messages. If the patient is offered the opportunity to participate but never calls back, there is a small chance that the person lost your telephone number but probably a greater chance that this nonresponse is a "soft no." You can make sure the patient has your contact information, be friendly, and answer any questions, but pestering the potential subject is not ethical or effective in the long run. The best indicator of effective recruitment is subject retention.

Study Visit Tips

Study visits with research subjects are conducted in hospitals, in clinics, and in the community. They typically are carried out face to face and by telephone, although social networking is beginning to make its way into research recruitment activities. Many clinical studies do not involve human subjects. In these types of studies, "the subject" may be a catheter tip, a hospital room, or a piece of medical equipment. No matter where or how study visits are happening, some key considerations should be kept in mind:

- The safety of subjects, clinical staff, and research personnel is always the primary consideration. Clinical trial visits are usually conducted in a clinic or hospital setting with readily available emergency personnel and equipment. Research personnel, like their clinical colleagues, use *personal protective equipment* (PPE) and follow precautions to protect themselves from exposure to blood-borne pathogens, infectious diseases, and other occupational hazards. Compliance with institutional policies and national regulations for the safe handling and shipping of research specimens protects research staff and the public.

- Site personnel need to understand all the timing considerations when scheduling and conducting study visits. It is not just about whether a study visit time will work for the subject and research team's schedule. For example, the central lab (the laboratory that processes all the specimens for every research site) may not be open to receive specimens on Sundays, so a Saturday study visit (where the specimen is shipped out for overnight delivery to the central laboratory on Sunday) is not feasible. The subject who works the night shift may prefer a 6:30 a.m. study visit, but the pharmacy, which dispenses the investigational drug, and the clinic, where the study-visit activities will be, may not open until 9:00 a.m. By thinking through the logistics, you can identify these and other barriers and try to work through them. For example, delivery of frozen shipments will require enough dry ice on hand to hedge against the possibility that the transport will take 2 days instead of the usual 1 day. The pharmacy and clinic may be willing to open early for the study visit. Clinical personnel may not always be able to accommodate research requests, but a case can be made for customer service. Research personnel should respect the existing clinical infrastructure and work through the proper channels with their requests to modify logistics.

- Depending on the type of trial and what needs to be done, research personnel may "roam" to meet with subjects, pick up specimens, or train research staff at participating sites on new procedures. Sometimes referred to as going on "field trips," research staff may travel for data or specimen collection or education.

- Research staff need to comply with their licensing requirements and practice regulations. If roaming is a part of the employees' job descriptions, research staff can check with their human resources department for answers to any questions about liability and worker's compensation they may have.

- If research personnel are planning to meet with a subject in another institution (e.g., hospital, nursing facility), they will need to work with the administration of that institution to secure approval. Medical facilities are required to maintain documented credentialing for all their employees and all other affiliated personnel, such as research staff or students. The institution's administration will want to know the purpose of the research staff's entering the facility and receive a copy of the subject's informed-consent document. They will want to know the qualifications of the research staff and exactly what is going to be done. This may be a formal process, especially if the activities are expected to be ongoing, or informal, resolved with a verbal explanation and a copy of the informed-consent form. Formal approvals should be kept on file. Informal approvals should have an NTF entered that documents the process kept in the research file.

- The study protocol may include planned telephone study visits. Research personnel may also follow up via telephone to check on subjects' status when an adverse event has occurred or to remind subjects about upcoming study-visit appointments. Typically the IRB will want to approve telephone scripts when site staff are providing study information to potential subjects. Research personnel are responsible for documenting all telephone communication with the research subject. Approach a telephone study visit with the same care and planning as if the subject were coming in to the clinic. Clarify the purpose of the telephone call and what needs to be accomplished. Is this a scheduled follow-up only, or do you also need to clarify information that was previously collected, such as concomitant medications or medical history? Be sure to have the protocol, the subject's source document binder, and the site-visit log handy during the call. Review the subject's record to refresh your memory about that person's study participation and events that have happened so far. Use a sponsor template or a visit checklist your site has created to note what is discussed during the telephone conversation.

EXAMPLE

A federally funded trial was conducted to determine whether genetic host factors predisposed a subset of patients affected by the West Nile Virus (WNV) to neuroinvasive disease (Loeb et al., 2011). The enrollment goal was 852 Nebraska residents who had tested positive for WNV. The study activities included collecting a blood specimen for genetic testing and retrieving medical-record documentation of the signs and symptoms. The study funding for research staff included 1.7 full-time employees (FTEs).

WNV is a reportable disease, and the incidence of cases clearly showed pockets of affected residents in rural areas in the middle and western portions of the state. The main study site was located in the eastern part of the state, and it was approximately an 8-hour drive from one end of the state to the other.

A plan was needed to recruit and consent subjects, manage the communication and documentation on each subject, collect and ship the specimens, and, based on the clinical documentation, designate whether each subject had neuroinvasive disease.

For the recruitment plan, the investigator worked collaboratively with the Nebraska Department of Health and Human Services (DHHS), which agreed to send an IRB-approved letter to the persons affected with WNV in staggered mailings. The letter explained the study and invited interested persons to call a toll-free number if they were interested in more information or participation.

For the informed-consent process, the investigator obtained IRB approval for a telephone-consent process. A team approach was implemented, having research assistants receive the telephone calls and the CRC conducting the informed-consent process.

For communication and documentation, the research staff developed an intake form to document the incoming callers' contact information, a file system for each subject's records, the consent and medical record, and an Access database to efficiently manage the high volume of contacts and to create accurate counts for the reports.

For specimen collection, the investigator contracted with a company that provided services for health-insurance physicals that included

continues

blood-specimen collection. This company's personnel were located throughout the state and traveled to each subject's location for collection of the blood samples. Courier services were arranged with a company that had dropoff locations throughout the state.

The study was a success. The Nebraska study site was on time and met the enrollment target of 852 subjects. The 1.7 FTE was divided into 1.2 FTE for research assistant and outsourced phlebotomist support and 0.5 FTE research nurse coordinator support. The research assistants handled incoming calls, sent out consent and medical release forms, filed paperwork, created a database, and completed data entry and data queries. The research nurse coordinators supported the regulatory documentation and telephone consents and set up the subject charts for the investigator's review. By having a clearly defined process and steps for each of these activities, the research staff could keep up a steady pace and shift effort to other tasks when bottlenecks occurred.

> **TIP**
>
> *When considering which materials will be needed for the screening visit, the research staff can create a supply of "ready-to-roll" folders containing several copies of the informed-consent form (one for the subject and extras in case the patient brings a family member to the visit), the investigator's business card, and information about research participation and the subjects' rights. The research staff may also plan to bring other IRB-approved items to support the explanation of the study, such as a calendar or an electronic diary device.*

Many protocols have scheduled milestone study visits. The purpose of these visits is often to assess subject safety and to gather study-specific data. These data may be as simple as taking the subject's vital signs (measuring blood pressure and temperature for example), collecting blood specimens, or following a patient's medical procedure. In addition to conducting study visits, the investigator and research personnel are processing regulatory documents, screening and recruiting potential research subjects, and entering the subject data into the sponsor's database.

> **TIP**
>
> - *Prepare for upcoming study visits by looking at the next day's schedule or pulling up the schedule for the upcoming week.*
>
> - *Some other ideas may include placing appointment reminder calls to the subjects, pulling their source documents, and reviewing what exactly will need to be done and what needs to be clarified when they come in at the time of the visit.*
>
> - *If specimens are going to be collected, check on whether there are enough collection kits and that the supplies are not expired.*
>
> - *Check to make sure the clinic visits are on the schedule and any orders are entered.*
>
> - *If the subject will be given new specimen collection supplies at the time of the study visit, then now is the time to make sure you have them.*
>
> - *Having a shelf to set up the study visit materials for each subject may be helpful.*

If research personnel are planning to meet with their research subject in another institution (e.g., hospital, nursing facility), they will need to work with the administration of that institution to secure approval. Medical facilities are required to maintain documented credentialing for all their employees and all other affiliated personnel, such as research staff or students. The institutional review board (IRB) for the institution may require documentation of what is being done.

The institution's administration will want to know the purpose of the research staff's entering the facility and may request a receive a copy of the subject's informed-consent document. They will want to know the qualifications of the research staff and exactly what is going to be done. This may be a formal process, especially if the activities are expected to be ongoing, or informal, resolved with a verbal explanation and a copy of the informed-consent form. Formal approvals should be kept on file. Informal approvals should have a note to file (NTF) entered that documents the process kept in the research file.

The study protocol may include planned telephone study visits. Research personnel may also follow up with their research subjects via telephone to check on how they are doing when an adverse event has occurred or to provide reminders about upcoming study-visit appointments. Typically the IRB will want to approve telephone scripts when site staff are providing study information to potential subjects. Research personnel are responsible for documenting all telephone communication with the research subject. Approach a telephone study visit with the same care and planning as if the subject were coming in to the clinic. Clarify the purpose of the telephone call and what needs to be accomplished. Is this a scheduled follow-up only, or do you also need to clarify information that was previously collected, such as concomitant medications or medical history? Be sure to have the protocol, the subject's source document binder, and the subject visit log handy during the call. Prior to making the call, review the subject's record to refresh your memory about that person's study participation and events that have happened so far. Use a sponsor template or a visit checklist your site has created to note what is discussed during the telephone conversation.

Specimen Collection

Many clinical trials involve collecting specimens for research testing. Investigators and their research staff collect the samples or retrieve the results from clinical testing. The same standards that apply to clinical laboratory specimens (i.e., accurate patient identification and specimen labeling) apply to research samples. Because study specimens are critical to the outcome of a clinical trial, study personnel must adhere to the protocol specimen-handling procedures and documentation. In addition, specimens must be handled according to laboratory and shipping policies and regulations to protect study and clinical personnel as well as members of the public.

A local laboratory may be part of the investigator's institution or the laboratory that provides clinical services for the investigator's patients. Research personnel must comply with their laboratory's policies and procedures. The research coordinator or assistant is responsible for research specimens from the point of collection to the point of delivery to the local laboratory.

The sponsor may use a designated laboratory, sometimes called a central laboratory, to process all the study specimens for such reasons as standardizing the testing and controlling expenses. This means shipping the biological samples. The International Aviation Transportation Association (IATA) regulates the transportation of dangerous goods under the authority of the International Civil Aviation Organization (ICAO) and the U.S. Department of Transportation. Research personnel must complete the training for shipping and comply with their institution's policies and procedures.

The sponsor makes shipping arrangements with a specific courier, such as Federal Express, United Parcel Service, or World Courier. Major couriers have websites and processes for delivery pickups and tracking shipment status. Billing is usually handled directly between the study sponsor and the courier, and study-site personnel are informed of the account numbers to use.

> **TIP**
>
> *Research personnel working in a clinic examination room collect specimens from the research subject during the study visit. They transport these specimens in a rigid, leak-proof container to a laboratory area where they will be processed according to the research protocol and packaged according to IATA regulations for shipping to the central lab.*

Copies of the shipping airbills and other declaration documents need to be maintained in the investigator's research files in the event of issues during transport. One filing option is to create a shipping reference binder that contains shipping airbill copies, reference information about the regulations, and training documentation for the research staff. Site staff may also file copies of the shipping airbills in the subject's source document binder, but a general shipping binder that has all the information in one place is very helpful for audits.

The study sponsor, IATA authorities, and investigator's institution will have guidance on how long shipping documents need to be maintained. An auditor is typically going to ask to see all the shipping documents for the shipments made in the previous 6 months.

Specific information about the proper handling, packaging, and storage of specimens and supplies is included in the study protocol. Storage includes maintaining the protocol-recommended temperature ranges for ambient, refrigerated, or frozen specimens.

> **TIP**
>
> - *Existing laboratory policies at the investigator's institution can be referenced for the research Standard Operating Procedures (SOPs). The investigator can provide additional specific research-related details for the SOP, such as which personnel are responsible for collecting and processing the research specimens; specimen transportation methods using leak-proof, rigid containers; and the research site's process for review of results as appropriate.*
>
> - *When specimens are provided to a central laboratory, the research protocol will identify the time that the specimen is viable, specimen transportation logistics, and processes for procuring supplies.*
>
> - *Shipping refrigerated or frozen specimens involves maintaining and documenting temperature control (the cold chain) for the specimens. Dry ice, a solid*

form of carbon dioxide, is commonly used as a cooling agent for shipping refrigerated or frozen items. When the dry ice pellets thaw, they change from a solid to a gas—hence the name "dry ice." It is important to declare the contents of shipping boxes containing dry ice, as the carbon dioxide may build up in confined environments, such as airline cargo holds. Personnel handling dry ice should don protective gloves to avoid frostbite. Sometimes specimen temperatures during transport are documented using thermometers that maintain a record of the temperature or change color when a temperature ranges beyond a set range. The receiver is responsible for reading the device and documenting that the temperature remained constant during shipping.

- *A research laboratory's records should include a detailed inventory of all equipment that specifies the item, serial number, and current location. In addition, user manuals, purchasing documentation, and equipment-calibration records are important to maintain in the files.*

- *Research personnel are responsible for documenting temperature control of the refrigerators and freezers where investigational drugs, supplies, or specimens are stored. These items may not be stored together in the same equipment. Temperature monitoring can range from placing a thermometer in the unit and manually noting the readings on a log sheet all the way to a sophisticated continuous monitoring system that activates an alarm if temperatures vary too greatly. The investigator must know the acceptable ranges for the materials being stored as well as what is to be done with the specimens when temperature excursions occur. In some cases of temperature excursion, a quality control check may be sufficient, but in others, the materials may need to be sequestered until their viability can be determined.*

Administration of Study Medication

Clinical research trials may involve outpatients who self-administer the study medication. In these situations, the investigator and research staff are responsible for working within their institution's pharmacy system to dispense the research medication and to teach the research subject how the investigational drug is administered. When clinical research trials involve inpatient research subjects, the investigator, research staff, or clinical nursing staff may administer the investigational drug within the institution's pharmacy system.

> **TIP**
>
> *A good source of guidance on medication administration may be your institution's nursing policies. For example, the nursing guidelines likely reference such practices as using two patient identifiers, such as the name and date of birth, to verify a patient's identity.*
>
> *Also, nursing professionals follow the principles of the five "rights," which means the right drug, at the right dose, at the right time, by the right route, and to the right patient.*

Clinical research staff are responsible for understanding and complying with their institution's pharmacy policies.

Activities After the Study Visit

After the subject has left and the specimens have been dropped off or shipped to the laboratory, the next set of tasks revolves around documentation. The protocol usually includes a reference to the sponsor's goal for the completion of the study data entry: that it be done as soon as possible. The study monitor will have access to the database to read the documentation and may issue queries. The database may have "logic" programmed into the system and auto-query when out-of-range values, dates, or conflicting information is entered.

CHAPTER 6: Managing Clinical Trial Activities and Processes 147

Follow-up activities include making copies of relevant information from the subject's medical record; updating tracking forms, such as the subject-visit log; claiming or monitoring the flow of site charges for protocol-related medical tests into the grant account; and processing stipend payments, if applicable.

> **TIP**
>
> *At the time of data entry, look over the entire source document binder to check for other information that needs to be entered, such as the resolution dates on concomitant medications, adverse events, or medical history updates. Make sure documents are filed in the correct sections in preparation for the next monitoring visit.*

Ways to organize information to complete a case report form (CRF) or eCRF include the following:

1) Gather protocol, sponsor guidelines for CRF completion, and the subject's source document binder for reference.

2) Retrieve relevant medical records from the chart and/or electronic record. If requesting records from another institution, fill out and get the request form signed. Review records received against the records requested.

3) Read and sort the subject's documents in the medical record, separating unrelated records from those related to the current patient encounters or study-related illness. Keep key records that document medical history, discharges, or clinic summaries by printing or creating an electronic report.

4) Find confirmatory testing and laboratory results in the study-visit source documentation or medical record.

5) Print copies of the investigator's review of results for the investigator to date and sign. The sponsor may want the investigator to also note whether results are CS, for clinically significant, or NCS, for not clinically significant. Equivocal results can be provided to the investigator for guidance.

6) Complete CRF pages.

7) Check the electronic system for queries and resolve them as soon as possible.

Organizing the Administrative/Clerical Workflow

The other aspects of organizing the clinical trial workflow are managing the administrative and clerical tasks. The same critical thinking skills and triage mind-set in the clinical setting are just as valuable for research personnel when working on research documentation.

Triage starts with identifying tasks and activities that are of high priority. One way to start the day's activities is to create a paper, electronic, or mental list of what needs to be done. Once listed, the tasks can be prioritized and reprioritized as the day goes on. Staying on top of the priorities is key to keeping things organized and on track.

Check schedules, messages, and reminders. Think in terms of what needs to be done this morning, what needs to be accomplished by the end of the day, and what will need to be done tomorrow and by the end of the week. Consider how individual tasks relate to future activities.

> **EXAMPLE**
>
> *A clinical trial evaluating disinfection practices for intravascular catheter hubs evaluated differing lengths of time spent cleansing the catheter hub (Rupp et al., 2012).*
>
> *The preparation for collecting the samples included drafting a short protocol describing the processes for collecting the specimens. A data-collection form needed to be developed along with a short "elevator speech" to use to explain the study to patients. In addition, such supplies as alcohol wipes and growth media plates had to be ordered, and research laboratory personnel had to be scheduled. After a "rehearsal" of the entire process, the study was ready to start.*

Research involves many variables beyond the control of the investigator and the research personnel. For instance, it may take weeks to get institutional review board (IRB) and sponsor contracts approved. The investigator and their staff must precisely follow the clinical trial protocol. Recruitment and screening activities may be unscheduled and occur outside of an 8:00 to 4:30, Monday through Friday work week, as the availability of potential subjects in acute care settings is often unpredictable.

The good news is that many aspects of the study are under the control of the investigator and site personnel. Research personnel can use critical-thinking skills to identify distracters and time wasters in the work environment.

- Does your workspace face the door? If so, then everyone who walks by will be distracting and lead to interruptions. Unless greeting incoming subjects is part of your responsibilities, consider rotating your work area or partially closing the door.

- Many times, the workspace for research personnel is limited. Consider ways to create "invisible walls" around the desk space. Listening to music through earbuds may help some people focus, but, as a member of the research team, you should not be totally unaware of your surroundings. Recognize and respect your co-workers' concentration levels and personal workspace by minimizing personal conversations and batching questions whenever possible.

- Working through e-mail alone can consume the entire day if allowed. Does your computer make a sound every time a new e-mail message comes in? This feature can be turned off. If you are a "message junkie," wean yourself to checking e-mail every 2 hours, then every 4 hours. Or set small goals, such as waiting to check e-mail until after finishing a specific task or study visit.

- Consider ways to sort research documents. It is challenging and a huge time waster to search for specific documents stacked in a giant pile. One way to solve this problem is to first identify some categories within a study, such as regulatory and each individual subject's study documents, and place them into three-ring binders or a file. You might create a regulatory binder with sections for the different document types. If the regulatory binder has a section for IRB communication and you know that this section alone will contain hundreds of pages, one option is to make a *note to file* (NTF) stating the IRB communication is located in its own binder, which could be titled "Study Name XXX IRB Communication."

- Next consider how to make the documents for each clinical trial easier to identify. The use of colored paper and pictures is inexpensive and provides visual relief in the virtual sea of words and documents involved in the clinical trial. Inexpensive colored file folders can be assigned to a specific study. A study-specific logo or picture makes it easy to quickly separate stacked items on a desk. Once you have a logo or picture, it is simple to create a coversheet or spine using desktop publishing that contains the IRB number, study name, and binder purpose.

Three-ring binders with page pockets on the cover and spine come in all sizes, are lightweight, and are reusable when a study is complete. This printed cover page and spine can be easily created and slipped into the cover and spine. The binders stack neatly on a shelf and can be quickly grouped using the logo and name, and the documents stay in their proper section until needed.

A simple strategy for labeling each binder includes the nickname of the study, perhaps the IRB number, and the specific purpose of the binder (e.g., "Study Communication" for all study-related correspondence filed in date order, "IRB Communication" for all IRB correspondence filed in date order, or "Screening" containing the specific pages with inclusion and exclusion criteria and all the screening logs). The use of clip art can create some levity, but remember to make professional choices and recognize that the binder cover may be seen by clinical personnel or research subjects. A skeleton may seem like an ideal logo to consider if you are doing a clinical trial for osteoporosis, but if your subjects are very elderly, they may interpret this image as a reference to death.

Sometimes each study or the research subjects participating in the study may have relatively few documents, so simple file folders with inexpensive metal anchors can hold the information.

- Consider ways to keep productivity up throughout the workday. Spending an entire day making phone calls, filing paperwork, or writing regulatory guidelines can become very tedious. Accuracy with redundant tasks, such as data entry, can diminish after a short period of time. So consider breaking up data entry into several short sessions throughout the day.

> **EXAMPLE**
>
> *The investigator's community-based clinical trial site had 852 subjects (Loeb et al., 2011). The essential documents in each subject's source documents were the original signed consent form, several pages of documentation of telephone conversations between the subject and study staff, and several pages of the specific medical records needed to document the subject's relevant medical condition. Even the smallest three-ring binder would have taken up limited research office space, so the research staff used inexpensive blue file folders with anchors to secure the papers inside the file.*
>
> *The individual file folders were inexpensive, easy to work with, and easy to distinguish from other studies' documents and easily stored in locked cabinets in the investigator's research offices.*

If you focus best in the early morning, reserve an early morning time slot for drafting regulatory documents. Generally speaking, making telephone calls to subjects during the daytime may not be successful if subjects are working or out of their houses and away from their home telephones. You may be much more successful at reaching them later in the afternoon or early evening, or the subject may have a cell phone.

Research tasks can also be sorted. One way to do this is to categorize them by frequency: daily, weekly, monthly, quarterly, or annually. By keeping an eye on activities that fall beyond today, the groundwork can be laid for upcoming commitments. One way to keep essential tasks top of mind is to create a Study Reminder Checklist (see Form 6.3).

FORM 6.3 Study Reminder Checklist

Frequency	Task	Activity/document type
Daily		
	Check messages	Phone and email
	Temperature monitoring and documentation for research specimen or supply refrigerators or freezers	• Maintain temperature log on front of equipment. • File log in the regulatory binder.
	Carry out screening and recruitment activities.	• Use the study-specific inclusion/ exclusion criteria as a worksheet. • Communicate with referral sources.
	Conduct a high-level review of each clinical trial or project.	• What is happening? • What needs to be done? • What are we waiting to hear about or finalize?
Weekly		
	Check subject-visit log for each study for upcoming study visits.	• Verify accuracy of dates. • Update all current and estimated future dates.
	Conduct subject study visits.	• Complete source document checklists.
	Perform data entry.	• Check electronic database for queries and resolve. • Enter new data.
	Check supplies.	• Blood-collection kits • Office supplies
	Attend investigator update meeting.	• Update agenda with discussion items. • Update spreadsheet of current studies.
	Prepare for next week's meetings.	• Set up file folder. • Insert relevant documents. • Review attendee list. • Create agenda, including relevant items for discussion or decisions. • Send agenda to meeting leader or attendees as appropriate.
	Review and clear out email messages.	• Download electronic correspondence and place into intermediate filing.
	Do final filing.	• Choose one trial or project to do complete filing on.
	Check milestones.	• Check clinical-trial recruitment status: goals, screened, enrolled. • Check on upcoming deadlines for PI projects.
Monthly		
	Scheduled reports	• Complete reports.
	Check schedule for quarterly milestones	• Recruitment status on each clinical trial • Regulatory milestones • PI project deadlines
Quarterly		
	Reports	• Expect routine monitoring visits. • Update quality-control documents for each study. • Get recruitment status on each clinical trial. • Check regulatory milestones. • Verify PI project deadlines.

> **TIP**
>
> *Being unprepared for a study visit when a subject arrives, miscalculating or missing a study-visit window, having expired collection supplies or incomplete visit logs, being months behind on subject stipend payments, and using an outdated consent form are all examples of problems that can be avoided through the use of organizational and time-management tools.*

Documentation and Reports

Protocol-related activities for an inpatient study may include review of the subject's status in the electronic medical record by checking on clinical progress notes, medical orders, and laboratory and test results. The research nurse coordinator can go on "rounds," or bedside visits on the clinical unit, to have the opportunity to speak with the clinical caregivers about how the subject is doing and to update them on study activities in progress. The research nurse coordinator can also evaluate the research subject and communicate with the IP for investigational drug-dosing logistics. After these activities, the coordinator can provide a report to the investigator. The protocol will detail the study activities at each milestone visit. See Form 6.4, Schedule of Events (also reviewed as Form 3.2 in Chapter 3).

The research nurse coordinator is usually responsible for the completion of the source documentation and will make notes and retrieve or create the reports for each subject's research chart. If the investigator's institution has electronic medical records, paper reports can be printed, but they should also contain an electronic notation or the signature and date of the research personnel retrieving this record. Sponsors may ask for a "certification" of the printed records and will define what they would like to have recorded besides the signature and date. Sponsors will want the study monitor to verify the printed records against the electronic records. The monitor will also check for the omission of any relevant records.

FORM 6.4 Schedule of Events

	Screen	Visit 1 D1	Visit 2 D8	Visit 3 D15	Visit 4 D22	Visit 5 D29
Window plus/minus	minus 2	0	1	1	2	2
Study visit-clinical	X	X	X	X		
Study visit-telephone					X	X
Informed consent	X					
Medical History	X					
Concomitant Medication	X					
Physical Examination	X	X		X		
Body weight	X			X		
Vital signs	X	X		X		
12 lead ECG [a]	X					
Pregnancy test	X	X				
Echocardiogram	X	X				
Randomization		X				
Study drug administration		X	X			
Study diary		X	X	X	X	X
Safety laboratory tests [b]	X	X		X		
Stool sample [c]		X	X			
Adverse Events		X	X	X	X	X
Key:	a) local test		b) central laboratory			
	c) site to store and batch ship to central laboratory					

Such documents as laboratory test results should be signed and dated by the investigator when they are reviewed.

Financial Reports

The budget, reconciliation of test charges, study payments, and grant accounts are usually reported in monthly, quarterly, and annual cycles. In many cases, members of the research team work collaboratively with their institution's finance personnel to contribute the detailed information needed to arrive at a true picture of the site's finances. For example, the PI's financial administrator likely works in the institution's finance and grant accounting systems. The research coordinator is working on individual studies. The investigator has a true picture of study status when dollars from the finance administrator's perspective and data from the research coordinator's perspective are combined.

Progress Reports

Some sponsors will create periodic progress reports and require the study sites to provide data at milestone points during the study. For example, the clinical trial contract for federally funded trials usually clearly identifies the PI's reporting responsibilities. At the start of the study, the investigator and support personnel should carefully review these reporting obligations and create the plan for the who, what, when, where, and how of getting this done.

> **EXAMPLE**
>
> *A federally sponsored trial had a total of six participating research sites running under the oversight of one PI. The PI was responsible for submitting monthly, quarterly, semiannual, and annual reports to the sponsoring agency that included information on enrollment status and financial expenditures, such as payroll, travel expenses, and supplies. The secondary investigator at each site was responsible for submitting data to the primary site in a timely manner for these reports. The secondary investigator and staff worked collaboratively with the PI to create a data report in formats for the primary site to add to the master report.*

Correspondence

Over the course of the study, the sponsor's monitor will document site visits and findings and maintain reports in the sponsor's files. The monitor will send official correspondence to the investigator to confirm meeting dates, times, and a short description of what will be reviewed, such as the regulatory binder and subject source document files. The monitor will send follow-up letters to the investigator after the visit to document findings. This correspondence must be maintained in the study site's regulatory files.

Other relevant correspondence includes letters (paper or electronic) between the sponsor and investigator, meeting notes, and notes made about telephone calls between site, sponsor, and research subjects. One option for filing this documentation is to maintain a communication binder where all correspondence is filed in date order.

Keep track of the primary care physicians referring or caring for your research subjects and provide them with information about the clinical trial to promote continuity of care and patient-centered communication. The IRB may require documentation of the communication between the investigator and primary caregivers regarding subject recruitment.

Communication tools, such as a Clinical Trial Summary (see Form 6.5) or advertisements and flyers with study information for subjects will need to be approved by the IRB.

Research Team Communication

Team communication is vital, of course, but determining the content, context, and frequency of communications is dictated by the type of clinical trials and the makeup of the research team. Daily or "real-time" communication makes the most sense for critical or urgent issues. For instance, the PI needs to know about adverse events, serious adverse events (SAEs), and protocol deviations as soon as they are identified by any member of the research team.

Based on the protocol, the PI or secondary investigators may not necessarily be present at every study visit. The CRC and research assistants may carry out the visit tasks, and an advanced practice nurse may perform the physical examinations. Then, an e-mail containing the study updates can be sent to and acknowledged by the investigator and filed in the subject's source document binder. This is a simple way to document the communication process within the study team and demonstrates that the investigator is fully aware of the subject's safety and status. Another option is to incorporate routine subject updates into the weekly update meeting with the PI. Bottom line: The PI needs to be aware of subject safety and study status.

FORM 6.5 Clinical Trial Summary

Title of Trial	*Effectiveness of chlorhexidine gluconate (CHG) general skin cleansing in reducing the occurrence of catheter-associated bloodstream infections and the transmission and/or infection rate due to multi-drug resistant organisms in hospitalized patients.*
IRB Number/Approval	*xxx*
Name of Trial	*CHG Bathing Study*
Investigator	*Mark E. Rupp, MD*
Coodinator	*Name: Jen Cavalieri, BSN, RN, CCRC, CCRP*
	Telephone: *Pager:*
Purpose of Study	*The purpose of this study is to determine the effect of daily bathing with a dilute solution of chlorhexidine gluconate on the rate of intravascular catheter-associated infections and the rate of acquisition/transmission or infection due to specific micro-organisms.*
Enrollment Goal	*All patients hospitalized, with the exception of neonates and newborn nursery patients.*
Study Duration	**Start:** *16 February 2009* **End:** *August 2011*
Procedures	• *Chlorhexidine (CHG) bathing will be introduced first to patients in the ICU areas.* • *For the first 6 months, CHG bathing will be done on Mondays, Wednesdays, and Fridays. After the initial 6-month period, CHG bathing frequency will increase to daily.* • *At the 3-month milestone, CHG bathing will be introduced to the remainder of patients in the hospital on a Monday-Wednesday-Friday schedule. After 6 months, the CHG bathing frequency will increase to daily.* • *The Investigational Product is stocked in the supply machines on each unit. Staff will remove product for their patients on a daily basis. There is no patient charge.* • *Patients and parents of pediatric patients are advised to use the CHG with bathing/showering by applying the product from the neck down.* • *Research staff will be collecting monthly census and bottle usage data* • *Patients may decline to bathe with the CHG product.* • *Adverse events will be monitored by notifications from the clinical staff and/or the hospital incident reporting system.*
Possible Risks	• *Extensively used for several decades* • *Dermatologic reactions: no evidence of absorption, low potential for reactions* • *Case reports of hypersensitivity, anaphylaxis, ototoxicity, corneal injury are rare*

QUESTIONS? Contact *Jen Cavalieri, Research Nurse Coordinator*
Phone here - Pager here - Email here

> **TIP**
>
> *Daily updates and reporting among front-line research team members make sense. The research nurse coordinator is responsible for many details and activities. The investigator and other members of the research team expect reports on outcomes or problems, not necessarily a blow-by-blow listing of the details.*
>
> *Research-staff activities may include setting up tomorrow's study visits, assembling specimen-collection supplies and restocking expired items, completing documentation after the study visits on the subject logs, processing stipend payments, and making copies and assembling research consent or source document binders. None of these routine activities may be necessary to report to the investigator.*

Weekly Updates

Weekly reports are a productive use of time for the PI and a lead CRC. They can review study progress and plan for upcoming study milestones and related activities. A simple spreadsheet can list current trials and projects, logistical issues, and related responsibilities, such as research training or education (see Form 6.6). The spreadsheet can serve as a template that is updated weekly, which makes setting up the report efficient. Notes can be made on each week's report about the PI's decisions and action items for the CRC to follow up on.

Weekly or monthly meetings can be useful for research teams with multiple coordinators and research assistants. These meetings provide opportunities for announcements and high-level reviews of active trials that affect the majority of staff. It is helpful to stay focused on high-level details and provide more specific information as needed.

FORM 6.6 Weekly Report

	Status	Notes
Study A	Open, 3 active subjects/3 completed subjects	• Data Safety Monitoring Board meeting Friday • Potential subject in screening
Study B	Pending, regulatory, and contract approval in progress	• Working on source documents • Micro lab meeting Tuesday
Study C	Open, 12 active, 24 completed, 2 screen failures	• Monitoring visit Wednesday and Thursday • Protocol amendment coming • Monthly coordinator conference call Monday
Project #1	Week 4 of 6, total hubs sampled = 340	• Repeat lab cultures • Draft abstract for deadline 01 OCT 12
Time	Holiday 24 NOV 12	• CRC out 24–25 NOV 12 • PI on call and will cover active subjects

> **TIP**
>
> *Communicate with the department manager when placing flyers on bulletin boards or in waiting rooms. Many options for reaching inpatients, outpatients, and visitors to the institution can be ethically carried out.*

Study Closeout

Every clinical trial comes to an end. The research protocol identifies the number of study subjects, and enrollment ends when the final subject is randomized. The clinical-trial activities continue until the final study visits are completed.

In some cases, the sponsor may reassess the analysis and preliminary results to determine whether the original number of subjects can be revised and still reach the study endpoints. Or subject accrual may be dismally below expectations. In this case, the sponsor may consider revising the protocol or closing the study early.

When the final subject is enrolled at a research site and the date of the final study visit is known, the investigator and research personnel should start thinking about several things, such as:

- Reconciling sponsor payments
- Preparing regulatory documents for study closeout
- Transitioning effort to a new trial
- Consolidating and organizing documents in preparation for long-term storage

For industrial studies, the results may take a year or more from the final study visit before they are released. Investigator-initiated or federally sponsored trials may not take as long.

> **EXAMPLE**
>
> *The cath hub study (Rupp et al., 2011) was designed in response to questions from clinical personnel about the adequacy of catheter disinfection. The data were gathered over a 6-week period of time, and results were provided to the clinical staff within 8 weeks. This type of rapid-cycle feedback is valuable, but for many clinical trials, it may take years before the results are known.*

The investigator should inform their referral sources and clinical stakeholders when the study is completed. A common complaint is that after the study closes, these people never hear about the study's outcome. Investigators who want their help on future studies should make every effort to provide results to these referring clinicians and other interested parties.

Key Take-Aways

- Adopting a systematic approach to managing study visit–related activities, study documentation, and communication will enhance productivity.
- Workflow of clinical and administrative tasks happens simultaneously; therefore, organizational strategies for each is necessary.

Suggested Reading

Fedor, C. A., Cola, P.A., & Pierre, C. (2006). Responsible research: A guide for coordinators. London: Remedica.

References

Cavalieri, R. J. (2003a). Recruiting strategies for clinical trials; Lessons learned from practice. *Applied Clinical Trials Magazine, 12*(1), 44–58.

Cavalieri, R. J. (2003b). Effective advertising strategies for clinical research sites. *Clinical Researcher, 3*(5), 12–17.

Loeb, M., Eskandarian, S., Rupp, M., Fishman, N., Gasink, L., Patterson, J., . . . & Lemire, M. (2011). Genetic variants and susceptibility to neurological complications following West Nile Virus infection. *Journal of Infectious Diseases, 204,* 1031–1037.

Rupp, M. E., Yu, S., Huerta, T., Cavalieri, J., Alter, R., Fey, P., Anderson, J. (2012). Adequate disinfection of a split-septum needleless intravascular connector with a 5-second alcohol scrub. *Infection Control and Hospital Epidemiology, 33*(7), 661–665.

Chapter 7
Managing Data and Research Records

Managing study data and documentation may seem daunting and tedious. This chapter demonstrates ways that research personnel can effectively manage their study information by providing ideas for creative tools and templates and identifying professional habits to cultivate. The goal is to collect sound study data and transfer this raw data into a useable system. New and experienced research personnel may benefit from ideas on how to do this efficiently.

Research Roles and Responsibilities

The *investigator* is responsible for the integrity of the research data and the physical and electronic security of the research records. *Research coordinators*, *assistants*, and *regulatory specialists*, working under the direction of the investigator, perform the day-to-day regulatory support, data collection, and documentation of clinical trial data.

A *study sponsor*, the source of funding, develops the protocol and arranges for research sites to generate the data needed to answer the research question. The sponsor has overall responsibility for the trial and should employ qualified personnel to handle and validate the data, perform the analysis, and write and submit the trial reports.

> **TIP**
>
> *Expect the sponsor to conduct extensive prestudy evaluations when selecting participating research sites. Starting up a research site is a considerable financial investment for the sponsor.*

Monitors are sponsor representatives who are responsible for the review and validation of the study data. They visit the research site regularly and will spend hours to days reviewing the subject data and regulatory files. Monitors are trusted resources when protocol questions arise.

Data

Data are the information gathered for the research study. Data can be a research subject's blood pressure, symptoms, or chest X-ray result. The organization and management of data are critical to any trial.

Data Integrity

Research professionals commonly use ALCOA guidelines that were first introduced by the Federal Drug Administration (FDA). ALCOA stands for "attributable," "legible," "contemporaneous," "original," and "accurate."

Attributable refers to the clear identification of who documented and edited the data.

> **TIP**
>
> *Corrections to data are made with a single strikethrough, noting initials and explanation as needed. Never try to obliterate the original data, as doing so creates questions about what the original data indicated. Simple human errors occur, but it is always necessary to preserve the data trail.*
>
> *A Site Staff Task Delegation Log (see Fpr, 7.1) usually contains the site personnel's initials as a reference for the person who made the corrections.*

FORM 7.1 Site Staff Task Delegation Log

Name of site staff	Study role	Tasks	Start	End	Initials	Site staff signature	PI signature
Mark E. Rupp, MD	Principal investigator	1.2.3.4.5.6.7. 8.9.10,11, 12, 13,14, 15, 16, 17, 18	04AUG10		MER		
	Secondary investigator	1, 2, 3, 4, 5, 10, 11	04AUG10				
R. Jennifer Cavalieri	Lead study coordinator	2, 8, 12, 14, 15, 16, 17, 18	04AUG10		RJC		
	Investigational pharmacist	6,7,9	04AUG10				
	Research assistant	16,17	04AUG10				
	Laboratory assistant	15	04AUG10				

Legible handwriting is a reasonable expectation in every practice setting.

Contemporaneous refers to documentation at the time the event occurred. Source documents should be completed at the time of the study visit so that valuable data are not lost due to memory issues or unexpected absence of the study personnel. The data entry of source document information should be completed as soon as practical.

Original refers to the source of the documentation. This may be the research investigator's electronic documentation of their findings from the physical examination of the subject, the CRC's handwritten notation of the subject's blood pressure on a visit checklist, or the subject's study diary notes.

Accuracy refers to telling the whole truth during a trial. Deliberate falsification of data is fraud. Missing data or failure to perform protocol-specific procedures are study violations.

Data Ownership

The ownership of the research data is specified in institutional policies and sponsor contracts. Any transfers of ownership may also involve regulatory authorities.

Research personnel or students working on a clinical trial under the direction of the investigator do not own the data they collect, although they may be compensated in the form of a salary and authorship.

Research investigators working on industry-sponsored drug or device trials may have limited or, in most cases, no claim to any intellectual property related to the product being developed.

Retention of Study Data

The length of data retention depends upon the type of study. This will be specified in the sponsor's contract, investigator's institutional policies and guidelines, and federal requirements. Expect to see differences between what is required for an investigator-initiated trial versus a clinical drug or device trial.

The Food and Drug Administration's (FDA) approval process for investigational drugs and devices can take many years. This means the study records will need to be retained in a secure manner for a significant period of time. The research site is responsible for costs associated with record retention.

The investigator should understand the institution's storage options, whether the storage is on site or off site, and related fees, such as the annual storage rate and charges for box retrievals.

Documentation

Documentation in research is the evidence or source of the study-related information. Some examples of typical documentation found in a clinical trial are a patient's medical record, source documents, CRFs, individual research subjects' study information in binders or files, and tracking and sign-in logs.

Source Documents

Source documents are the original source of information located in medical records, which can include X-rays or scans, or public records, such as death certificates. Also, source data may be created at the time of the study visit when study staff measure vital signs and record the results. A Screening Visit Checklist (see Form 7.2) is a useful tool for sites to create as a task reminder and an appropriate place to record data and comments. It is important to record every study visit or conversation with a research subject. If information or test results are missing, document their absence. Supply all information requested and do not leave blanks on pages.

Research personnel may jot down hasty notes, such as vital signs on a paper towel or the back of a hand. In the case of the former, the paper towel can be attached to the subject's research record. The latter, the hand issue, could be resolved by photocopying the hand with the information and attaching the paper to the record. However, the study monitor or an auditor will likely find this habit problematic at best. Research personnel should cultivate professional documentation practices instead. Creating site-specific checklists for study visits in the subject source document binder is very useful for reminding personnel of typical visit activities, recording data, and making notes.

FORM 7.2 Screening Visit Checklist

Date: _____ Time: _____

VITAL SIGNS BP _____ Temperature _____ C / F Pulse _____ Respirations _____

MEDICAL HISTORY yes   **CONCOMITANT MEDICATION HISTORY** yes   Weight _____

PI PHYSICAL EXAMINATION yes   date _____   print dictated report

ALLERGIES _____   **ECG** yes date _____ (w/in 28 days prior to randomization)

LABORATORY

Serum Pregnancy Test yes Result: _____   no   reason: _____

Blood (Central Lab) Collection date _____ time _____ centrifuge time _____ shipped yes no _____

ECHOCARDIOGRAM

Scheduled Date _____   Time _____

Clinical procedure per hospital protocol.   Data collection and de-identified CD of procedure:

Report of Results: _____   PI Review _____

STUDY DIARY

Education _____

STUDY DRUG

Education _____

SPECIMEN

Collection supplies: Kit   Cool pac (store in freezer)   Instruction sheet   labels

DAY 1 APPOINTMENT

Date _____   time _____   clinic room scheduled

Urine collection cup for pregnancy test Visit 1 DAY 1   Collection supplies   Instructions

Randomization of Study Drug by Investigational Pharmacist **Scheduled Pick Up** _____   **Date** _____   **Time** _____

Medical orders (specimen collection, pregnancy test) into medical record

TRACKERS

Subject Visit Log   Master Subject Log

Coordinator: _____   Date _____

A research subject may be given a study diary and instructed to note the date and time the investigational drug is taken. If the subject decides to note the date and time the investigational drug was taken on the top of the medication box instead, research personnel can attach the medication box top to the diary and reinstruct the subject to use the diary for future documentation. Because the "original" information was documented on the box top, the subject or research staff should not redocument the medication dates and times onto another form. Research staff should make a comment or note to file (NTF) that explains why the documentation was recorded this way. Some sponsors or IRBs might consider this unconventional documentation to be a study violation, because the diary was not used. If the information was not recorded anywhere, then that would likely be considered a study violation.

Case Report Forms

Source document data are recorded by research personnel onto Case Report Forms (CRFs). The sponsor, or the investigator when conducting an investigator-initiated trial, creates CRFs on paper, in electronic web-based systems called electronic Case Report Forms (eCRFs), or in spreadsheets created with Excel, Access, or SAS.

The sponsor, or in the case of investigator-initiated studies, the investigator and the biostatistician, analyze the study data entered into the data systems.

Note to File

A useful method for clarifying events or issues is to create a *note to file* (NTF). Research personnel should strive to maintain thorough, accurate study documentation and use the NTF option only when necessary. Some typical uses might be to track relocation of documents or to explain unusual events.

A NTF should describe the who, what, when, where, and why of the event details and corrective action steps, if indicated. Additional essential information to include are the author of the documentation, the date that the NTF is being written, and an identifier, such as the protocol name or IRB number that ties it to the clinical trial. The site may print the NTF on institutional or department letterhead.

Source Document Binder

One option for organizing the source documents for each subject is to create a source document binder or file (see Table 7.1). This concept is similar to the way a patient's essential medical records are assembled in a paper or electronic chart. Research personnel can certainly set up electronic subject files or paper folders. The binder strategy makes it easy to keep the subject-specific information organized and portable enough to take from the investigator's research offices to the study-visit locations in the clinic or inpatient unit. Documents in this binder include copies of selected medical records, data-collection forms, and tracking spreadsheets. The subject's *electronic medical record* (EMR) and the source document binder are companion references about the subject. The data in the patient's EMR, the source documents, and the research CRFs/eCRFs should all match.

FORM 7.3 Source Document Binder Contents *(customize this with study-specific information)*

Section	Description	Comments and tips
Front	Study Schedule of Events (SOE) (Shown in Chapters 3 and 6)	Readily available for reference. Recommendation: If the sponsor has not created one, or if this is an investigator-initiated trial, it is well worth the time for site personnel to create this.
	Demographic information	Print the medical record fact sheet listing name, contact information, next of kin, etc. OR Create a form and fill in this information
	Original signed informed-consent form and documentation of the process (Shown in Chapters 5 and 7)	This all-important document can be maintained in the subject's source documentation or filed in the study regulatory binder
	List of target study visit dates and/or calendar	Study-visit calendars are easy to create by going online and downloading a free blank template. Generally a monthly view works well. Placing 3 months on a page provides a valuable at-a-glance view of upcoming target visit dates.
	Site Visit Log (Shown in Chapters 4 and 6)	This log is useful for review of enrollment status, upcoming visits, and compliance validation.
	Stipend payments (Shown in Chapter 3)	This log is useful for tracking the stipend payment process.
Screening section	Inclusion and exclusion worksheet	This may be provided by the sponsor or can be created by copying the protocol into a new document. This is very useful to make notes on as subject eligibility is confirmed, and it should be signed and dated by the investigator.

CHAPTER 7: Managing Data and Research Records 171

Section	Description	Comments and tips
	Site-Specific Screening Checklist (Shown in Chapter 7)	Customized checklists help research personnel keep track of study-specific tasks.
	Medical and medication records that support subject eligibility and medical condition	Could include medical records, notes made by the investigator from the physical exam, or study staff interviews with subject.
	Investigational Drug Talking Points (Shown in Chapter 7)	Education worksheets listing talking points with subjects about completing the study diary, administration of the investigational product, or what to report to study personnel Research personnel can check off each item as it is addressed and make notes.
Randomization section	Copies of the documentation received (e-mail or fax) noting the subject and/or drug randomization	
Section for each visit 1–5	Site-specific visit checklists	
	Physician documentation	Dictated summaries of subject status, physical examinations, and communication with the medical monitor and sponsor
	Copies of specimen requisitions, shipping airbills, and tracking confirmation	Specimen requisitions may have stickers on the form that are to be attached to the specimen containers and the site record form or spreadsheet.
	Laboratory reports (signed, dated and noted as clinically significant [CS] or not clinically significant [NCS] by investigator)	One option is to keep the laboratory reports with the study visit information. Another option is to create a study-specific tab where all laboratory results are filed.
Concomitant medications	A listing of all medications of interest for the study. The protocol often defines the time period of interest, such as the previous 12 months, previous 7 days, etc.	This documentation could include medication references in admission or discharge summaries, medication administration records (MARs) from the patient's medical record, or a spreadsheet created by the sponsor or site personnel with such key information such as the name, dosage, frequency, and start and stop dates.
Echocardiogram	Sponsor instructions for specific data collection	
	Report results and any relevant medical orders	
Adverse event section	Subject tracker for AEs	Keeps track of adverse events of interest for the study. Allows for review of types, onset, and resolution of the events.
Serious adverse event section	Subject tracker for SAEs (Shown in Chapter 5)	Keeps track of report dates to the IRB and sponsor, onset, and resolution of the events.
	Each adverse event can be its own subsection and contain documentation from when the SAE was first discovered through IRB and sponsor notification, request for information from the sponsor's safety professionals, query resolution and additional information, and completion of the site documentation.	Keeps detailed documentation of the related information.

> **EXAMPLE**
>
> *If the Screening Visit Checklist contains a note about a specimen-collection time that does not match the time on the specimen requisition form or in the EMR, the discrepancy must be explained. Any number of things could have occurred: Maybe the phlebotomist could not successfully access a vein at the first attempt and time lapsed until the collection was completed, perhaps the research coordinator confused military-time notations, or a simple transcription error could have occurred when the requisition form was completed. If the reason for the discrepancy cannot be explained, the NTF can doument this.*

Once the study source document binder has been created, keep one as a template and make one or two more for use when the first few subjects are enrolled. There will likely be changes to the forms or organization of the binder once they are road-tested, so setting up more than a few binders initially is usually not a good use of time. Once you have a reliable working set of forms, create a supply of binders for "grab-n-go." An assembly line to create six at once is much more efficient than making up single binders as needed. It is a good idea to have as many of the enrollment-related tasks completed ahead of time as possible.

Creating Documentation Tools

Research personnel can develop such tools as the source documents Screening Visit Checklist (see Form 7.2), and Investigational Drug Talking Points (see Form 7.4), to manage the daily operations at the research site.

The first step to creating a source document Screening Visit Checklist is to consider what needs to be done and what the natural flow of events during the visit will be. Assemble key references, such as the detailed protocol, schedule of events (SOE) page, and your site recruitment plan. Your knowledge of the resources and how things work at your site also factor in to creating this tool. This process helps identify the unknown details of how things work at the site. It is important for research personnel to use the time prior to enrolling the first subject to clarify specific processes.

> **EXAMPLE**
>
> *Gaps in logistics and study procedures can be identified and corrected with a little forethought. For example, the protocol states that the study specimens will need to be sent to the sponsor's designated central laboratory. The sponsor's designated courier comes to the investigator's institution, but the study staff does not know the internal pick up locations and time. The research staff can "rehearse" the logistical steps prior to the first subject's being enrolled and draft a process. Consider your drafted process to be a work in progress, as the process and documentation tools will be refined while working with the first few subjects.*

FORM 7.4 Investigational Drug Talking Points *(customize with study-specific information)*

IRB#	Study
Site Investigator:	**Subject ID Num**

Date

The study drug is in capsule form. 1:2 chance of placebo (no active drug)

The study drug needs to be started 1 day after the screening visit.

The first dose will be administered during your research visit appointment. You need to take the remaining three doses for the day at noon, 6pm, and 10pm. Show the subject the written instructions on the study drug package.

Do not open or crush the capsules. Swallow the capsule whole using any beverage you wish. There are no study-related food or beverage restrictions.

It is very important that you keep the empty study drug bottle. Please bring this with you for your next study appointment.

It is very important for you to note the time you take your study drug in the diary. Always bring your diary with you for your study appointments.

If you forget to take your medicine at your regular time, skip that dose and take the next regularly scheduled dose.

Your next appointment is scheduled for _____. You will receive the study drug for that day at that study visit.

Call your study nurse at XXX-XXX-XXXX if you have any questions

Coordinator: Date:

Most studies start with subject screenings, during which potential subjects and the investigator will discuss the study opportunity, and if the patient is interested and meets the study criteria, the detailed informed-consent process (ICP) can begin.

The Screening Visit Checklist can include reminders and places to make notes about the ICP. Another option is to create a separate, simplified Informed Consent Documentation Tool (see Form 7.5) for documenting some of the activities related to the ICP, such as notes about the subject's questions and reminders for research staff about key tasks. However, the tool is not intended to replace the investigator's documentation of the ICP.

FORM 7.5 Informed Consent Documentation Tool

DATE (DD-MMM-YYYY):

The process of informed consent was conducted at _____ on _____ prior to the start of any study related procedures	Individuals present:
Questions asked by the patient and answered by the research personnel:	
Consent type	adult proxy:
Copy of signed consent form given to subject	yes no Reason:
Copy of Subject Rights Education given to subject	yes no Reason:
Copy of consent placed in medical record	yes no Reason:
Progress note in chart	yes no Reason:
Consent version used:	

Research Coordinator: _____ Date: _____

So, once ICP is completed, other screening-visit activities can be performed. While customizing the checklist, do a mental walk-through of the process and specific steps involved at your research site. See the Schedule of Events (shown in Chapter 3 and 6) for a sample list of activities. The checklist provides reminders and places to document this information. Sections for study diary and study drug education include spaces for the research coordinator to make comments, or more detailed lists of talking points can be created.

As this visit ends, activities for the next appointment can be listed as a reminder for the research staff. For example, because the investigational pharmacist (IP) needs to randomize the subject, the research coordinator needs to communicate with the IP about this process. The research personnel responsible for administration of the investigational product need to schedule the pickup and maintain custody and the cold chain until administration. Each of these items is noted on the screening checklist in the section for the next appointment.

Some caveats about reminder checklists include the following:

- There is always the possibility of errors with omission of important tasks. In addition to the study checklists, keep the research protocol and Schedule of Events (SOE) page on hand at all times for reference.

- When using the checklist, do not leave blanks. If a task is on the checklist, it needs to be completed and checked off or addressed with a comment.

- Make sure the study-specific subject identification number, a unique identifier that does not disclose personal identifying information about the subject, the signature of the person making the notations, and the date are on every checklist.

- Once a checklist is created and used with the first few subject visits, improvements can easily be made.

Strategies for Organization

It is possible to maintain the printed documents in an organized manner. In fact, it's a must if the investigator is going to conduct efficient and budget-friendly clinical trials.

Communication

There are many types of research documents, ranging from correspondence from the sponsor to a subject's medical test results, for the investigator to review. Despite the move to electronic documents, investigators may still have many printed documents in their workspace. A simple strategy to implement is to use a specific color file folder for research documents so the investigator can quickly differentiate research from clinical documents. Color coding for a study is another effective strategy when the investigator is conducting multiple clinical trials.

Intermediate Filing

A tremendous amount of research communication is handled via e-mail. All study-related communication must be retained in the study files. An e-mail mailbox is not a filing cabinet. Electronic mailboxes have finite space, so these e-mails need to be filed with the study documents. Sorting, saving, printing, and filing each individual e-mail can be very time consuming. By batching the tasks of first downloading the messages, then sorting them by study, the e-mail box or incoming paper documents can be placed into an intermediate file. As you can imagine, filing each individual document into four separate studies is less efficient than sorting the pages into study specific "piles" and then filing all the specific study documents at the same time. Options for the "piles" can be a box or hanging file folder.

Holding boxes can be purchased from an office supply store, or any size sturdy box can be recycled and labeled with the study name and IRB number. Instead of boxes, study personnel may use a hanging file as a holding area for documents to be filed.

> **TIP**
> - *Time spent on communication and filing is usually not acknowledged in the study budget. Experienced investigators understand that this type of study effort must be factored in to the budget if the study is going to "break even," or have expenses meet revenue.*
> - *File regulatory documents and subject-specific documents immediately.*
> - *One option is to attach documents that have action items to the outside of the binder with oversized rubber bands as a visible reminder to complete those tasks.*

Reusable Supplies

Binders, folders, divider tabs, and plastic sleeves are all reusable. These items take up unnecessary space in boxes and are expensive to replace. When packing a completed study for long-term storage, remove these items and use oversize rubber bands and the binder cover page to keep the paper documents organized.

Key Take-Aways

- Valid research requires accurate and reliable data. The whole purpose of clinical research rests on producing or collecting data to answer the research question.
- There is no substitute for due diligence in clinical research and managing the data and research records.

Suggested Reading

Norris, D. (2009). Clinical research coodinator handbook (4th ed.). Medford, N.J.: Plexus.

Chapter 8
Professional Development

We hope you have found this guidebook to be a helpful source of ideas for your research practice. At this point, you may be wondering what the "next steps" and options are for professional development or process improvements. Every successful, professional leader, no matter what type of position held, actively pursues professional development opportunities. In this chapter, we present information about developing professional reading and presentation skills and networking with colleagues.

Next Steps

One way to start is to look for opportunities to learn within your organization. Academic medical centers are filled with teaching professionals. Asking questions is an excellent way to demonstrate interest and connect with someone who can provide answers or identify resources for finding answers. And you will certainly find that there are many questions with unknown answers. These may even lead to your next clinical research trial!

Journal Clubs

Reading and understanding professional journal articles is a worthy skill to be developed. Journals are printed or electronic periodicals that contain current articles or commentary on professional topics, such as research, and are published for a specific group, such as medical professionals or research personnel. A journal for professional nurses may contain articles about nursing interventions, clinical outcomes, or nursing research. A journal for research professionals may contain articles about regulatory, ethical, or good clinical practice (GCP) topics.

Your research group, department, or institution may already be holding journal clubs. The purpose of journal clubs is to learn how to critically review professional journal literature, to keep abreast of major developments through publications, to improve professional practice, and to have fun while learning from colleagues. If you find there are no journal clubs for research at your institution, start one! Gather interested persons for a brief planning meeting and identify the topics or the journals of interest. Schedule some dates and have each person choose an article to present.

One way to develop critical thinking and journal article review skills for beginners is to make some notes on a summary sheet, such as the following (see Form 8.1), while reading the journal article. Ask yourself these questions as you sort through the information in the article. This summary sheet can be useful for a quick review just before the journal club session begins.

FORM 8.1 Journal Article Summary Sheet

Title of article	Why is this topic of interest to the reader? Why was this article selected?
Author	Who are they? Where are they from? Any obvious conflict of interest?
Study goal(s)	Is this article worth reading? Find the goals to determine whether the article is relevant to the reader.
Figures and tables	• Go to these after you have clarified the study goals.
	• Find the table that describes the study subjects. This will contain some demographic data, such as male-female, etc. Is there a clear balance of the baseline characteristics between groups?
	• How many subjects were involved in the study? (Subjects being a relative term— the subjects may be sampled objects, patient rooms being studied, etc.) If there is a small number of subjects, randomization may not equally distribute subjects. If it is a very large trial, randomization should result in an equal distribution of baseline variables (similar baseline demographics, underlying co-morbid conditions, etc.).
	• The figures/tables should also give you some sense of the "generalizability" of the article.
Any evidence of bias or confounding variables?	Bias is when an outcome is favored as a result of a sampling or testing error.
	Confounding or extraneous variables may mislead an investigator into thinking that correlations exist. In research, it is challenging to remove extraneous variables.
Statistics	Efficacy = the difference in outcome between groups
	Find the reported "confidence interval," which indicates the magnitude and precision of the study. How big are the groups? Data with 95% confidence intervals (CI) are usually reported. Some people feel that 80% is sufficient.
	P value is an indicator of how likely it is that your outcome is due to chance. P values are arbitrary, but generally 0.05 is regarded as a cutoff point. • $p < 0.05$ means there is a statistically significant difference. • $0.05 < p < 0.1$ is a borderline statistically significant difference (trend). • $P > 0.10$ means there was no statistically significant difference.
Conclusions	Do you agree w/the author(s) concluding statements (based on the data and methods utilized)?
	Are other relevant events affecting the outcome/conclusions?

The person presenting the article can talk through the key points of the study and discuss any observations and opinions about the article with the others attending the meeting. During the remainder of the scheduled time, you may find that the discussion then moves to a dialogue with your colleagues about related examples and challenges. Journal clubs are a great chance to learn and connect with your colleagues during a lunch hour or in the early evening. Any journal club presenter will probably tell you he or she learned more from preparing for the meeting than by simply attending.

Research Posters

Research posters are commonly used to present initial research results at professional meetings. There are several ways to enhance the use of posters and make the most out of them at a meeting.

First, make sure to use the right venue. Identify a professional meeting that has an interest in your research topic. Check the submission rules and instructions carefully for information on the topics the meeting organizers are looking for. Identify and comply with instructions related to deadlines, poster types and size, and the schedule for when your poster will be displayed. Explore your logistical obligations and production costs. There may be support in the form of a waiver of the meeting registration fees if you are a presenter.

Next, make sure the approach and content reflects the poster purpose. Is the poster intended to teach or present findings to professional colleagues? Is the message clear and organized? Sections of the poster may contain the background, a brief description of the methods, the results, and conclusions or implications of the results. Choose professional and relevant graphics and pictures as well as a simple layout style for your poster. Avoid too much text, and the text size should be readable from 6 feet away. Make prudent use of "white space" to enhance eye appeal and attract attention. Graphs should be simple, demonstrate data patterns, and highlight key results.

Posters are usually displayed in a large room that has many visual aids displayed on easels or boards. The event organizers may print a list of all the poster titles and authors so conference or event attendees with an interest in your topic can "find you." Thus, it is important to have a "catchy" title that attracts attention but does not misrepresent your findings. Dress professionally, stand to the side of the poster, and behave as if you are at an "interview." You have approximately 15 seconds to engage with your audience before they move along to the next poster. Provide an explanation of the poster contents while the audience is viewing the tables and graphs. Answer questions and take note of your audience's comments for use after this event. Attendees often appreciate receiving a page-sized reproduction of the poster. Lastly, to reach an even broader audience and more permanently document your findings, develop the poster content into a journal manuscript.

Watch for opportunities to do this at upcoming events that will have a poster session. If you do not have enough time or information to proceed with your own poster, attend the event and network with some of the poster presenters about their preparations and experience. This will help you be prepared to create your own poster for the next event opportunity.

Professional Associations

Two large organizations for research professionals are the Association for Clinical Research Professionals (ACRP) and the Society of Clinical Research Professionals (SoCRA). Their websites, www.acrpnet.org (ACRP) and www.socra.org (SoCRA), contain information about the organizations, such as their annual conferences, continuing education opportunities, and certification programs. Each of these groups also has a network of local chapters that research professionals can use to connect with local colleagues.

Busy work schedules and economic constraints can make continuing education and attending national conferences challenging or out of reach. Members often create a local chapter for exactly these reasons.

A large organization will provide contact information for local chapters and guidance for individuals who are interested in starting up a new local chapter. The professional organizations charge annual membership dues and will have specific policies on what the local groups can do to raise funds and the types of approved educational offerings.

Certification

Certification opportunities exist for such groups as research investigators, research coordinators, research monitors, and regulatory personnel. The certification process often involves the use of standardized testing to assess research knowledge and application of the knowledge as well as documented, relevant work experience. Maintenance of the certification may involve periodic retesting and a required amount of continuing education.

Preparing for a certification examination usually begins once a research professional has been working in the research specialty for a while. It can take up to 2 years for a new research professional to attain a strong working knowledge of the complex research tasks involved in the conduct of clinical research. Taking the examination then serves as a benchmark signifying practice competency. Once certification is achieved, the research professional can list the specific certification initials, or designation, after his or her name.

Fees are associated with preparing for and taking the certification examination. Maintaining certification status usually requires ongoing renewal fees and a significant level of continuing education. The professional organizations provide this information.

Some employers support the preparation course, examination and renewal fees, and time spent on continuing education. Some research groups require new employees to achieve certification within a designated period of time to maintain employment. Most of the time, however, pursuing certification is voluntary.

The benefits of certification for the research professional include a personal sense of achievement and satisfaction in meeting benchmarked research standards. It demonstrates a commitment to this specialized body of knowledge. Hiring managers and employers appreciate such benchmarks as certification when evaluating job applicants and job performance. Industry sponsors understand the rigor of certification and appreciate working with research sites that have certified research personnel.

Continuing Education

Many research professionals are already familiar with the need for ongoing continuing education in order to maintain their licenses or clinical obligations. Professional growth usually means doing more than just what is required. One strategy for solving clinical research challenges is to look "outside" customary educational avenues and develop skill sets from other disciplines that will complement or augment the research professional's professional abilities.

Some options might be to take some evening classes to improve writing or public relations skills. Short sessions aimed at improving computer skills may be offered at your institution. Developing proficiency with software, such as spreadsheets and desktop publishing, can be immediately put to use with financial management and recruitment materials.

> **TIP**
>
> - *Keeping track of continuing education and training may be necessary for licensing, employer, or certification purposes. One option is to maintain the relevant licensure and continuing education in a personnel file at work.*
>
> - *People are responsible for their own license and certification maintenance and need to develop a personal system to keep track of these documents.*
>
> - *Excel spreadsheets or log sheets can be easily created to track continuing education, annual clinical competencies, and education.*

Pop Quiz

Can you identify the mistakes represented by the following statements?

1) This new clinical trial is budgeted for $8,000 per subject. This sounds great!

   A sponsor's budget is only half the equation. How much will it cost for you to do the study? (Chapter 3)

2) I would like to work in research so I won't have any more evening or holiday work commitments.

   Research can rarely be contained in a Monday through Friday, 8:00am–4:30pm schedule without sacrificing outcomes. (Chapter 6)

4) Conducting a few clinical trials would be a good way to generate some revenue.

   Conducting a few clinical trials is a good way to lose money. (Chapter 3)

5) I need to recruit 20 research subjects. Please make 25 informational flyers for distribution.

   The screen-to-enroll ratio may be as low as 2:1 and higher than 50:1. (Chapter 6)

6) I want to do some clinical trials. I will split one of the clinic nurse positions, and they can spend half their time in the clinic and the other half as a research nurse.

> *Asking staff to balance competing priorities, such as clinical and research responsibilities, sets the "research" portion of the position up for failure. (Chapter 6)*

7) We only have two active research subjects. I wonder why my research nurse is so busy?

   Research coordinators are involved in almost every aspect of the daily operations for clinical trials. (Chapters 1–7)

8) We are too busy to create SOPs. Everyone knows what to do and what is expected of them.

   SOPs are the foundation for compliance, staff accountability, and orientation. (Chapter 2)

Closing Remarks

Every new clinical trial is an opportunity to utilize improved tools and processes and reach study outcomes more efficiently. We've learned the everyday "nuts and bolts" of clinical trial conduct the hard way, had plenty of missteps, and created unnecessary work for ourselves along the way. We hope others can have a smoother acclimation into research, avoid some common headaches, and run well-functioning, valuable, and self-sustaining clinical trials by reading this book and learning from our experience.

Key Take-Aways

- Research professionals are leaders and life-long learners.
- Extracting key information from a journal article and creating research posters are professional skills worth developing.
- Certification and continuing education are ways to expand professional skills and development.

Suggested Reading

Salka, J. (2005). *First in, last out: Leadership lessons from the New York Fire Department.* New York: Portfolio.

Appendix A

Your Go-To Regulatory Reference Tool

COMMON REFERENCE	WHO ARE THEY
CH Guidelines	The International Conference on Harmonisation (ICH)
Investigator Responsibilities	U.S. Department of Health and Human Services Food and Drug Administration Center for Drug Evaluation and Research (CDER) Center for Biologics Evaluation and Research (CBER) Center for Devices and Radiological Health (CDRH) Procedural (October 2009)
The CFR	GPO, U.S. Government Printing Office
Guidance for Institutional Review Boards	U.S. Department of Health and Human Services/FDA/ U.S. Food and Drug Administration
Informed Consent Guidelines	U.S. Department of Health and Human Services/FDA/ U.S. Food and Drug Administration
Electronic documentation and electronic signatures	U.S. Department of Health and Human Services/FDA/ U.S. Food and Drug Administration
Investigational new drug applications (INDs)	U.S. Department of Health and Human Services/FDA/ U.S. Food and Drug Administration
HIPAA Privacy Protections	U.S. Department of Health and Human Services

APPENDIX A: Your Go-To Regulatory Reference Tool

BACKGROUND	WEBSITE
The ICH was formed to develop unified standards for clinical trials so the clinical data can be accepted by the regulatory authorities for members. GCP is an international, ethical, and scientific quality standard for designing, conducting, recording, and reporting trials involving human subjects.	http://www.ich.org/products/guidelines
Guidance for Industry Investigator Responsibilities — Protecting the Rights, Safety, and Welfare of Study Subjects.	http://www.fda.gov/downloads/Drugs/
Code of Federal Regulations (CFR)	http://www.gpo.gov/fdsys/browse/collectionCfr.action?collectionCode=CFR
21CFR Part 56 Institutional Review Boards Office for Human Research Protections (OHRP) The Federalwide Assurance (FWA)	http://www.accessdata.fda.gov/scripts/cdrh/cfdocs/cfcfr/CFRSearch.cfm?CFRPart=56 http://www.hhs.gov/ohrp/assurances/irb/index.html http://www.hhs.gov/ohrp/ http://www.hhs.gov/ohrp/assurances/assurances/filasurt.html
21CFR Part 50 Elements of informed consent	http://www.accessdata.fda.gov/scripts/cdrh/cfdocs/cfcfr/CFRSearch.cfm?fr=50.25
21CFR Part 11 FDA criteria for acceptance of electronic records, electronic signatures, and handwritten signatures executed to electronic records as equivalent to paper records and handwritten signatures executed on paper	http://www.fda.gov/RegulatoryInformation/Guidances/ucm125067.htm
21CFR Part 312 Procedures and requirements governing the use of investigational new drugs	http://www.accessdata.fda.gov/scripts/cdrh/cfdocs/cfcfr/CFRSearch.cfm?CFRPart=312&showFR=1
The Health Insurance Portability and Accountability Act of 1996 (HIPAA) Privacy and Security Rules Compliance with these regulations was required as of April 1, 2003 and defined the circumstances for the disclosure of health information, referred to as Protected Health Information (PHI)	http://www.hhs.gov/ocr/privacy/

continues

COMMON REFERENCE	WHO ARE THEY
Research Sanctions	U.S. Department of Health and Human Services/FDA/ U.S. Food and Drug Administration.
Public listings of Clinical Trials	ClinicalTrials.gov
	A service of the U.S. National Institutes of Health
Laboratory Guidance	CAP – College of American Pathologists
	CMS.Gov Centers for Medicare and Medicaid Services
	U.S. Department of Health and Human Services/FDA/ U.S. Food and Drug Administration
FDA	U.S. Department of Health and Human Services/FDA/U.S. Food and Drug Administration

APPENDIX A: Your Go-To Regulatory Reference Tool

BACKGROUND	WEBSITE
FDA Debarment List The consequences of research misconduct, according to the 21CFR, can be debarment, or exclusion from practicing research for the development of new drugs, for a period of time that depends on the seriousness of the offense.	http://www.fda.gov/ICECI/EnforcementActions/FDADebarmentList/default.htm
An electronic registry of clinical trials for interventional drugs and devices provides essential publicly posted information about the study.	http://www.clinicaltrials.gov/
Clinical Laboratory	http://www.cap.org/apps/cap.portal
Clinical Laboratory	http://www.cms.gov/Regulations-and-Guidance/Legislation/CLIA
21CFR Part 58 Good Laboratory Practice For Nonclinical Laboratory Studies	http://www.accessdata.fda.gov/scripts/cdrh/cfdocs/cfcfr/CFRSearch.cfm?CFRPart=58
Information Sheet Guidance for IRBs, Clinical Investigators, and Sponsors --FDA Inspections of Clinical Investigators	http://www.fda.gov/downloads/RegulatoryInformation/Guidances/UCM126553.pdf

Appendix B
Keeping Track of Things

Throughout this manual, we have presented common research situations where forms can be useful as organizational tools. This is necessary because study sponsors (and internal and external regulatory authorities) will advise the site personnel on "what to do" but not "how to do it." The "what to do" is specified in a research protocol and includes things such as the schedule for study visits and exactly what data and specimens to collect. The sponsor expects site personnel to handle the myriad of details around the logistics of working with subjects, tracking key study dates, and making sure that grant account charges and revenue flows to the correct accounts—in other words, the "how to do it."

So now that you have a sense of the rationale and usefulness of the forms, we can support your work by providing some templates that are ready for you to adopt and customize. Many seasoned research professionals will repurpose their site forms from previous studies when they plan and set up a new study. Since you may be new to research, we are giving you a jump-start by providing forms which can be downloaded when you purchase your book through www.nursingknowledge.org. These forms were built on software that is very user-friendly. Hopefully, you will find these forms useful, and you will realize greater efficiency in your own clinical trials.

Clinical Trial Summary

Title of Trial	
IRB Number/Approval	
Name of Trial	
Investigator	
Coordinator	Name: Telephone: Pager:
Purpose of Study	The purpose of this study is to determine
Enrollment Goal	
Study Duration	Start: End:
Procedures	
Possible Risks	

Research Nurse Coordinator: NAME

Phone here - Pager here Email: here

Clinical Trial Summary

This form can be used to communicate the study essentials to clinical professionals.
Strive to keep the information brief and the document length one-page.

Title of Trial	*Insert official clinical trial protocol name here*	
IRB Number/Approval	*Insert site's IRB number/approval date here*	
Name of Trial	*Insert study nickname here*	
Investigator	*Insert investigator's name here. Avoid numerous names as it may create confusion about whom to call*	
Research Coordinator	**Name:** *Insert name here*	
	Telephone: *insert number, make sure phone message has options for caller if there is no answer such as a pager # or the hospital operator's number*	**Pager:** *most research coordinators have work pagers or work cell phones. Providing personal cell phone or home phone number is not advised.*
Purpose of Study	*Use 1 to 3 sentences to describe the study purpose. One option is to take the purpose description from the consent form.*	
Enrollment Goal		
Study Duration	**Start:** *insert date*	**End:** *insert estimated date or year*
Procedures	*Provide a summary list procedures or procedure related activities.* *Do not list items such as obtain IRB approval, perform data entry, and analysis.*	
Possible Risks	*List a summary of risks, their likelihood and potential severity*	

QUESTIONS? List a resource person or 24/7 contact number here
Phone here - Pager here Email: here

Insert a footer containing document name and version information to make it easier to find in the clinical research professionals electronic file. Adding a date helps avoid using an outdated version of the document

Study Name:
Study Site Number:
Key Contacts

Sponsor Company Name:
Company Address:

Medical Monitor
Name:
Phone:
Email:

Sponsor Project Manager
Name:
Phone:
Email:

CRO
Name:
Phone:

Lead CRA
Name of Study Monitor:
Phone:
Email:

CRO Regulatory
Name of Regulatory Specialist:
Phone:
Email:

Central Laboratory
Name of company:
Contact Person:
Office Phone:
Email:

Position:
Name:
Address:
Phone:
Fax:

Position:
Name:
Address:
Phone:
Fax:

Position:
Name:
Phone:
Email:

Position:
Name:
Address:
Phone:
Fax:

Position:
Name:
Address:
Phone:
Fax:

Specialty Clinical or Ancillary Area *(such as echo lab, outpatient clinic, or microbiology bench)*
Name of area/manager/key contact person:

Phone:

Study Name Here
Study Site Number Here
Key Contacts

This tool is useful to sponsor and research site personnel. Try to limit the list to the essential contacts, using one page and keep it updated so it is relevant.

Sponsor Company Name:
Company Address:
Medical Monitor
Name:
Phone:
Email:
Sponsor Project Manager
Name:
Phone:
Email:
CRO
Name:
Phone:
Lead CRA
Name of Study Monitor:
Phone:
Email:
CRO Regulatory
Name of Regulatory Specialist:
Phone:
Email:
Central Laboratory
Name of company:
Contact Person:
Office Phone:
Email:

Principal Investigator
Name:
Address:
Phone:
Fax:
Secondary Investigator
Name:
Address:
Phone:
Fax:
Research Nurse Coordinator
Name:
Phone:
Email:
Lead Study Coordinator
Name:
Address:
Phone:
Fax:
Investigational Pharmacist
Name:
Address:
Phone:
Fax:
Specialty Clinical or Ancillary Area *(such as echo lab, outpatient clinic, or microbiology bench)*
Name of area/manager/key contact person:
Phone:

Financial Document File/Binder

Table of Contents

Section Options	Types of Documents
Agreements	
Correspondence	
Budget	
Reconciliation	

Financial Document Binder

Table of Contents

This tool provides the site with a binder or file description of essential financial documents and a suggested method for organizing to easily locate the documents. These documents may be originals or copies. Additional persons at the investigator's institution may be responsible for the financial documents. Having redundant filing provides the investigator with a quick reference and fail-safe backup plan.

Section Options	Types of Documents
Agreements	*• Copies of all CDAs, CTAs* *• Principal Investigator signature page for all protocol versions*
Correspondence	*• All communication between sponsor and investigator* *• All communication between investigator's institution and investigator* *• All communication between investigator's institution and sponsor (may be maintained in the institution's central files)*
Budget	*• Budget exhibit from the contract* *• Investigator's worksheets* *• Reference documents on test and procedure costs such as protocol schedule of events, ChargeMaster prices*
Reconciliation	*• Investigator's workbook* *• All original receipts from site purchases* *• Documentation of sponsor payments* *• Itemized payment details* *• Investigator's institution's internal accounting systems*

This page intentionally blank.

Example of a Site Budget

Start up fee *Includes IRB fee*	$4000.00
Screen failures *Up to 6*	$1650.00
Stipend (per subject)	$ 300.00

Per Subject Payments

Screening Visit	$1650.00
Study Visit 1	$1200.00
Study Visit 2	$ 550.00
Study Visit 3	$1000.00
Study Visit 4	$ 550.00
Study Visit 5	$1000.00
Study Visit 6	$ 550.00
Study Visit 7	$ 500.00
Study Visit 8	$ 500.00
Study Visit 9	$ 500.00
Total	***$8000.00***

All numbers are imaginary and should not be used in any way outside of this example.

Example of Schedule of Events Form

Protocol Title here

	Screen	Visit 1	Visit 2	Visit 3	Visit 4	Visit 5
Day						
Window plus/minus						
Study visit-clinical *type of visit*						
Study visit-telephone *type of visit*						
Informed consent						

Key

local test

central laboratory

site to store and batch ship to central laboratory

Example of Schedule of Events Form
Protocol Title here

	Screen	Visit 1	Visit 2	Visit 3	Visit 4	Visit 5
		day	*day*	*day*	*day*	*day*
Window plus/minus						
fill in matching activities to study visit						
Study visit-clinical *type of visit*	X	X	X	X		
Study visit-telephone *type of visit*					X	X
Informed consent	X					
medical record documentation	X					
medication documentation	X					
Physical Examination	X	X		X		
medical tests	X			X		
laboratory tests	X	X		X		
adverse events monitoring	X					

list protocol activities here

Key

a local test

b central laboratory

c site to store and batch ship to central laboratory

	Example Budget Workbook		
	Labor (12 months, estimate for 10 subjects)		
1	labor PI @ X %		calculate using labor workbook page
2	labor PI @ Y %		calculate using labor workbook page
3	Research Coordinator @ Z %		calculate using labor workbook page
4	Estimated Labor subtotal	$ -	total of line items 1, 2, 3
5	*Per subject estimate on labor*		**Divide line item 4 by the estimated number of subjects**
6	Start Up Fee		it is suggested that investigator negotiate this as non-refundable
7	Protocol intake	$ -	calculate the amount of time/effort needed to get the new study process started
8	Site Evaluation Visit (SEV)	$ -	calculate amount of time spent with study monitor
9	Invesitigator Meeting	$ -	calculate the cost of a work day for research personnel attending the meeting
10	Regulatory Document preparation	$ -	calculate the amount of time/effort needed to get the regulatory documents submitted to the sponsor and IRB
11	Site set up	$ -	calculate the amount of time needed for plannig meetings, source document set up, sponsor training for GCP & eDOC systems
12	Investigational Pharmacy	$ -	investigational pharmacist start up fee
13	Long term storage	$ -	Short and long term storage costs at the research site
14	**Start Up subtotal**	$ -	total of line items 7-13
15	Ancillary		
16	Investigational Pharmacy	$ -	*Investigational pharmacy cost of storage, randomization, record keeping, dispensing*
17	Tests	$ -	calculate using a test workbook page
18	Laboratory-local testing	$ -	calculate using laboratory workbook page
19	Laboratory-central lab support	$ -	calculate using laboratory workbook page
20	Ancillary subtotal	$ -	total of line items 16-19
21	Subtotal of start up	$ -	item 14
22	Overhead	$ -	*Percent is determined by investigator's site policy*
23	**Total for start up**	$ -	
23	Subtotal of per subject cost	$ -	Item 5 and 20
24	Overhead		*Percent is determined by investigator's site policy*
25	Per subject cost		
	Pass Through Expenses		
26	Regulatory Fee for IRB process	$ -	*Fee is determined by investigator's IRB*
27	Stipend for subjects	$ -	*study specific amount*

	Example Budget Workbook		note: demonstration purposes only: all prices are imag...
	\multicolumn{3}{c}{Labor (12 months, estimate for 10 subjects)}	
1	labor PI @ X %	$ 15,000.00	
2	labor PI @ Y %	$ 6,000.00	
3	Research Coordinator @ Z %	$ 22,000.00	
4	Estimated Labor subtotal	$ 43,000.00	
5	*Per subject estimate on labor*	$ 4,300.00	
6	**Start Up Fee**		non-refundable
7	Protocol intake	$ 1,000.00	site questionnaire, review of protocol, study feasiblity
8	Site Evaluation Visit (SEV)	$ 400.00	monitor visit
9	Invesitigator Meeting	$ 1,000.00	PI, research coordinator
10	Regulatory Document preparation	$ 1,500.00	regulatory binder, IRB submission
11	Site set up	$ 1,000.00	plannig meetings, source document set up, sponsor training for GCP & eDOC systems
12	Investigational Pharmacy	$ 500.00	start up only
13	Long term storage	$ 600.00	
14	Start Up subtotal	$ 6,000.00	
15	**Ancillary**		
16	Investigational Pharmacy	$ 100.00	per subject, covers storage, randomization, record keeping, dispensing
17	Tests	$ 450.00	per subject
18	Laboratory-local testing	$ 1,150.00	per subject
19	Laboratory-central lab support	$ 95.00	per subject for collection, processing, shipping
20	Ancillary subtotal	$ 1,795.00	per subject
21	Subtotal of start up	$ 6,000.00	item 14
22	Overhead	$ 1,560.00	26%
23	**Total for start up**	$ 7,560.00	
23	Subtotal of per subject cost	$ 6,095.00	item 5, 20
24	Overhead	$ 1,584.70	26% for this demonstration
25	**Per subject cost**	$ 7,679.70	
26	**Pass Through Expenses**		
27	Regulatory Fee for IRB process	$ 3,000.00	investigator's IRB fee
28	Stipend for subjects	$ 300.00	per subject

**Effort Log
Example
2013 Calendar
Month Here**

Day	Study A	Study B	Study C	Study D	educ	Special Project	PTO/ Holiday	Admin	Day Total	Week Total
1										
2										
3										
4										
5										
total										
6										
7										
8										
9										
10										
11										
12										
total										
13										
14										
15										
16										
17										
18										
19										
total										
20										
21										
22										
23										
24										
25										
26										
total										
27										
28										
28										
30										
31										
total										

Effort Log
Example
2013 Calendar
Month Here

Day	Study A	Study B	Study C	Study D	educ	Special Project	PTO/ Holiday	Admin	Day Total	Week Total
1	2	1	1	2		3			9	
2	1	3	4	0.5					8.5	
3	3	1	0	2		1		2	9	
4	2	2	3	0.5	1	1			9.5	
5		2			4				6	
total									42	**42**
6									0	
7									0	
8	3	1		1		2			7	
9	2	1.5		4					7.5	
10	4	2	1	1					8	
11	5	2.5	1						8.5	
12							8		8	
total									39	**39**
13									0	
14	4								4	
15	3	2	1	2		2			10	
16	2		3	1				1	7	
17	3	3							6	
18	5	2	2						9	
19	2		2	6					10	
total									42	**42**
20	3								3	
21									0	
22	1	3	5	0	1				10	
23	2	4	0.5	1				1	8.5	
24	1	1	4	3		2			11	
25	2		2	2		1			7	
26	4	2	1						7	
total									43.5	**43.5**
27									0	
28									0	
28	3	4		1					8	
30	2	2	3	1					8	
31	1	5	2						8	
total									24	

207

Summary Subject Stipend Payments

	Subject 1		Subject 2		Subject 3		Subject 4		Subject 5		Subject 6		Total
	Date	Amount	Date	Amount	Date	Amount	Date	Amount	Date	Amount	Date	Amount	
Screening													
Visit 1													
Visit 2													
Visit 3													
Visit 4													
Visit 5													
Total													

Summary Subject Stipend Payments

	Subject 1		Subject 2		Subject 3		Subject 4		Subject 5		Subject 6		Total
	Date	Amount	Date	Amount	Date	Amount	Date	Amount	Date	Amount	Date	Amount	
Screening	6-Feb-12	$ 25.00		$ 25.00		$ 25.00		$ 25.00		$ 25.00		$ 25.00	
Visit 1	7-Feb-12	$ 25.00		$ 25.00		$ 25.00		$ 25.00		$ 25.00			
Visit 2	14-Feb-12	$ 25.00		$ 25.00		$ 25.00		$ 25.00					
Visit 3	21-Feb-12	$ 25.00		$ 25.00		$ 25.00		$ 25.00					
Visit 4	28-Feb-12	$ 10.00		$ 10.00		$ 10.00		$ 10.00					
Visit 5	6-Mar-12	$ 10.00		$ 10.00		$ 10.00							
Total		$ 120.00		$ 120.00		$ 120.00		$ 120.00					$ 480.00

Allows for at-a-glance review of all subject payments shows total paid out to date

Labor Worksheet

Activities	One Time	Study Maintainance	Per Subject Hour	Notes
Site Evaluation visit				
Feasibility w/chart review				
Regulatory Start Up Documents				
Investigator Meeting				
Set up site process & documents				
eDoc and GCP training				
Regulatory support				
Serious Adverse Event reporting				
Daily Screening				
Monitor Visits				
Query Resolution				
Study Visits Screening (to final visit)				
Study CloseOut				
subtotal				
Total Raw Hours				

Labor Worksheet

1	Activities	One Time	Study Maint.	Per Subject Hour	Notes
2	Site Evaluation visit	4			monitor interview & tour
3	Feasibility w/chart review	6			read protocol, create budget, retro chart review
4	Regulatory Start Up Documents	4			regulatory binder, IRB submission
5	Investigator Meeting	16			estimated 2-day meeting w/travel (total time out of office)
6	Set up site process and documents	16			planning meetings w/ancillary stakeholders, create source docs receive and inventory supplies
7	eDoc and GCP training	20			estimated hours based on protocol
8	Regulatory support		40		amendments, request for change, annual continuing review
9	Serious Adverse Event reporting		4		estimated 1 per subject
10	Daily Screening		250		1 hour per day x 5 days x 50 weeks, screen logs to sponsor
11	Monitor Visits		40		10 hours x estimated 4 visits
12	Query Resolution		20		estimated hours based on protocol
13	Study Visits Screening - visit 9			12	estimated hours based on protocol
14	Study CloseOut	12			regulatory, supply return, inventory and pack records for storage
15	Subtotal	78	354	120	this per-subject number of hours needs to be multiplied by the number of subjects expected in year 1 of the study
16	Total Raw Hours				552 = 27% FTE 27% FTE = $27,600
17		78	354	120	multiply this by employee cost (salary plus benefit amount)

*Reminder: The numbers here are for example only and do not reflect true costs or true effort hours.

Tests & Laboratory Tests

	Internal Reference Number	Volume	Inpatient Technical Fee	subtotal	Research Rate	Professional Fee	Other	Per Subject total
Tests								
subtotal								
Local Labs								
subtotal								
Central Labs								
subtotal								
Per Subject Total								

Example Tests & Laboratory Tests

note: demonstration purposes only; all prices are imaginary

Tests	Internal Reference Number	Volume	Inpatient Technical Fee	subtotal	Research Rate	Professional Fee	Other	Per Subject total
Local Labs								
ECG		2	$ 300.00	$ 600.00	$ 250.00	$ 200.00		$ 450.00
subtotal								**$ 450.00**
blood: chemistry panel		3	$ 395.00	$ 1,185.00	$ 425.00	-		$ 425.00
blood: hematology panel		3	$ 400.00	$ 1,200.00	$ 625.00	-		$ 625.00
Serum Pregnancy test		2	$ 235.00	$ 470.00	$ 100.00	-		$ 100.00
subtotal								**$ 1,150.00**
Central Labs								
Specimen collection/ processing/ storage		3	$ 100.00	$ 300.00	$ 75.00	-		$ 75.00
Dry Ice		1					$ 20.00	$ 20.00
subtotal								**$ 95.00**
Per Subject Total								**$ 1,695.00**

Investigational Pharmacy Services

	Fee	Notes
Start Up		

	Fee	Volume	Per subject total
Pharmacy Storage			
Kit randomization and documentation			
Dispensing fee			

Example Investigational Pharmacy Services					
note: demonstration purposes only: all prices are imaginary					
		Fee	Notes		
Start Up		$ 500.00	one time, site evaluation visit, study set up and documentation		
		Fee	Volume	Per subject total	
	Pharmacy Storage	$ 25.00	2	$ 50.00	
	Kit randomization and documentation	$ 40.00	2	$ 80.00	
	Dispensing fee	$ 35.00	2	$ 70.00	
				$ 200.00	

Sponsor Payment-Remittance Detail

Batch #		Name of Research Site:
Trial Number:	Site Number:	Investigator:

Subject ID Num   **Payment for**   **Amount Due**

Sponsor:

Trial Number:

Payment Remittance

Name of Person at Research Site:

Research Site Address:

This page intentionally blank.

218

Payment Reconciliation Log

Protocol Title:

	Scr	Pmt from Sponsor	Visit 1	Pmt from Sponsor	Visit 2	Visit 3	Visit 4	Visit 5	Visit 6	Visit 7	Visit 8	Visit 9
Window plus/minus												
Subject #												

Example of Payment Reconciliation Log
Protocol Title here

	Screen	Pmt from Sponsor	Visit 1	Pmt from Sponsor	Visit 2	Pmt from Sponsor	Visit 3	Pmt from Sponsor	Visit 4	Pmt from Sponsor
			D1		D8		D15		D22	
Window plus/minus	minus 2		0		1		1		2	
Subject 2-0001										
Subject 2-0002										
Subject 2-0003										
Subject 2-0004	6-Feb-12	$ 1,650.00	7-Feb-12	$ 1,200.00	14-Feb-12	pending	21-Feb-12	pending	28-Feb-12	pending
Subject 2-0005										
Subject 2-0006										

a: local test; b: central laboratory; c: site to store and batch ship to central laboratory

Received	Date	Amount
Payment #1		
Payment #2		
Total Revenue to date		

date here	Total Revenue	
date here	Total Site Expense	

Research Personnel	Labor				Total to date
Date					
Principal Invest					
Secondary Invest					
Research Coord					
Total Salary to date					

Site Expenses	Expense				Total to date
Date					
ECG					
laboratory tests					
Invest Pharmacy fees					
Total Expense to date					

Received	Date	Amount
Payment #1	5-Jan-12	$ 22,500.00
Payment #2	3-Apr-12	$ 1,850.00
Total Revenue to date		$ 24,350.00

	date here	Total Revenue	$ 24,350.00
	date here	Total Site Expense	$ 16,533.32

Research Personnel	Labor					Total to date
	Jan-12	Feb-12	Mar-12	Apr-12	May-12	
Principal Invest	$ 1,250.00	$ 1,250.00	$ 1,250.00	$ 1,250.00		
Secondary Invest	$ 500.00	$ 500.00	$ 500.00	$ 500.00		
Research Coord	$ 1,833.33	$ 1,833.33	$ 1,833.33	$ 1,833.33		
Total Salary to date	$ 3,583.33	$ 3,583.33	$ 3,583.33	$ 3,583.33		$ 14,333.32

Site Expenses	Expense					Total to date
	Jan-12	Feb-12	Mar-12	Apr-12	May-12	
ECG		$ 300.00				
laboratory tests		$ 1,000.00				
Invest Pharmacy fees	$ 500.00	$ 400.00				
Total Expense to date	$ 500.00	$ 1,700.00				$ 2,200.00

IRB# ____-___-____
Study Title:
Site Name: **PI Name:**

Site Staff Task Delegation Log

Name of site staff	Study Role	Tasks	Start	End	Initials	Site staff signature	PI signature

Task Codes: 1-Informed consent, 2-Subject screening, 3-Physical Examination, 4-Evaluation of clinical laboratory testing, 5- Medical history, 6-Subject randomization, 7- Dispense investigational product, 8-Administer investigational product, 9-Investigational product accountability, 10-causality for AE(s)/SAE(s), 11- SAE reporting, 12-CRF/e-CRF completion and correction, 13-Review /sign off CRF/eCRF, 14- Query resolution, 15-Oversight of lab sample collection, processing and shipping, 16-Maintain study files, 17-Maintain regulatory files, 18-study budget   19-Other _____

IRB# XXX-yr-FB
Study Title here
Site Name here, PI Name here

Site Staff Task Delegation Log (example)

Name of site staff	Study Role	Tasks	Start	End	Initials	Site staff signature	PI signature
Mark E. Rupp, MD	Principal Investigator	1,2,3,4,5,6,7,8,9,10,11, 12, 13,14, 15, 16, 17, 18	04AUG10		MER		
	Secondary Investigator	1, 2,3,4,5,10, 11	04AUG10				
R. Jennifer Cavalieri	Lead Study Coordinator	2,8, 12,14,15,16,17,18	04AUG10		RJC		
	Investigational Pharmacist	6,7,9	04AUG10				
	Research Assistant	16,17	04AUG10				
	Laboratory Assistant	15	04AUG10				

Page __ of ___

Checklist for Regulatory Documents (TEMPLATE)

Study Name Here   IRB Number   Investigator name here
Research Coordinator: Jen Cavalieri

Submission Check List

Item	Submission	Response	Status	Note
IRB Application				
Request for Change				
Continuing Review				
P & T				

	Date signed	Fax to sponsor	Original to Sponsor	Comment
Original 1572				
PI signed				
PI signed				
Protocol	Date signed by PI	Fax to sponsor	Original to Sponsor	Reapproval date

	Version date	IRB approval	Sent to Sponsor	Comments
Adult Consent form				
PROXY Consent form				

INV Brochure		To Inv Pharmacist	To IRB

LAB	Expiration	Sent to Sponsor

Checklist for Regulatory Documents (EXAMPLE)   Study Name Here   IRB Number   Investigator name here
Research Coordinator: Jen Cavalier

Submission Check List

Item	Submission	Response	Status	Note
IRB Application v 1.1 16MAY11	19-May-11	3-Jun-11	conditional approval	
IRB Application v. 1.2 17JUN11	30-Jun-11	25-Jul-11	full approval	
IRB Application v.2.0 01APR12	5-Apr-12		approval	
Request for Change				
Administrative letter regarding change in XXX	3-Jan-12	10-Jan-12	acknowledged by IRB	
RFC Amend 1 02FEB12	6-Feb-12	20-Feb-12		
Continuing Review				
CR 1.0 02APR12	5-Apr-12	30-Apr-12	approval	
P & T				
IRB Application v 1.0 09MAY11	9-May-11	20-Jun-11		review date is 24MAY2011

Original 1572	Date signed	Fax to sponsor	Original to Sponsor	Comment
PI signed	19-Apr-11			local lab address does not match
PI signed	25-Apr-11		19-May-11	
Affiliation Note to File	26APR11		19-May-11	tie affiliated addresses to PI

Protocol	Date signed by PI	Fax to sponsor	Original to Sponsor	Reapproval date
Protocol 8888-100 version 10MAR11				
Protocol 8888-100 Amendment 1 version 02FEB12				

	Version date	IRB approval	Sent to Sponsor	Comments
Adult Consent form	v 1.0 16MAY11	conditional approval		sponsor approval 16MAY11
	v. 1.1 17JUN11		17-Jun-11	sponsor approval 28JUN11
	v. 1.2 29JUN11	25-Jul-11		
PROXY Consent form	v. 1.0 16MAY11	conditional approval		sponsor approval 16MAY11
	v. 1.1 17JUN11		17-Jun-11	sponsor approval 28JUN11

INV Brochure		To Inv Pharmacist	To IRB	
Edition 2 11AUG2010		9-May-11	19-May-11	
Edition 3 10MAY12		15-Jun-12	15-Jun-12	

LAB	Expiration	Sent to Sponsor
CLIA - Clinical Lab	19-Oct-12	5-Nov-10
CAP	23-Jul-11	4-Jan-10

IRB# XXX-yr-FB
Study Title here
Site Name here, PI Name here

Site Visit Log (template)

Sponsor Representative Name (printed)	Sponsor Representative Name (signed)	Date of Visit	Time Start	Time End	Visit Purpose	Site Personnel (signed)

IRB# XXX-yr-FB
Study Title here
Site Name here, PI Name here

Site Visit Log (example)

Sponsor Representative Name (printed)	Sponsor Representative Name (signed)	Date of Visit	Time Start	Time End	Visit Purpose	Site Personnel (signed)
Mary Smith, CRA		07MAY12	0900	1700	Site evaluation visit	
Betty Jones, CRA		30JUL12	0830	1730	Site initiation visit	
Betty Jones, CRA		10SEP12	0900	1715	Site monitoring visit	

Checklist for Regulatory Documents

Study Name: IRB Number: Investigator:
Research Coordinator:

Submission Check List

Item	Submission	Response	Status	Note
IRB Application				
Request for Change				
Continuing Review				
P & T				

	Date signed	Fax to sponsor	Original to Sponsor	Comment
Original 1572				
PI signed				
PI signed				

Study Name: IRB Number: Investigator:

Research Coordinator:

Submission Checklist

Item	Submission	IRB Response	Status	Note
IRB Application v 1.1 16MAY11	19-May-11	3-Jun-11	conditional approval	
IRB Application v. 1.2 17JUN11	30-Jun-11	25-Jul-11	full approval	
IRB Application v.2.0 01APR12	5-Apr-12		approval	
Request for Change				
Administrative letter regarding change in XXX	3-Jan-12	10-Jan-12	acknowledged by IRB	
RFC Amend 1 02FEB12	6-Feb-12	20-Feb-12		
Continuing Review				
CR 1.0 02APR12	5-Apr-12	30-Apr-12	approval	
Pharmacy & Therapeutics Committee (P & T)				
IRB Application v 1.0 09MAY11	9-May-11	20-Jun-11		review date is 24MAY2011

	Date Signed	Fax to Sponsor	Original to Sponsor	Comment
Original 1572				
PI Signed	19-Apr-11			local lab address does not match
PI Signed	25-Apr-11		19-May-11	
Affiliation Note to File	26APR11		19-May-11	tie affiliated addresses to PI

Protocol	Date Signed by PI	Fax to Sponsor	Comments	
Protocol 8888-100 version 10MAR11			Initial Submission Protocol	
Protocol 8888-100 Amendment 1 version 02FEB12			Incorporate change to inclusion criteria #5 and clarify storage of investigational product.	

	Version Date	IRB approval	Sent to Sponsor	Comments
Adult Consent Form	v 1.0 16MAY11	conditional approval	17-Jun-11	sponsor approval 16MAY11
	v. 1.1 17JUN11	25-Jul-11		sponsor approval 28JUN11
PROXY Consent Form				
	v. 1.0 16MAY11	conditional approval	17-Jun-11	sponsor approval 16MAY11
	v. 1.1 17JUN11	25-Jul-11		sponsor approval 28JUN11
INV Brochure		To INV Pharmacist	To IRB	
Edition 3	10MAY12	9-May-11	19-May-11	
Edition 2	11AUG2010	15-Jun-12	15-Jun-12	
LAB	**Expiration**	**Sent to Sponsor**		
CLIA - Clinical Lab	19-Oct-12	5-Nov-10		
CAP	23-Jul-11	4-Jan-10		

Subject Demographic Tracker
Name of Study

Total	Subject ID Num	Sex		Ethnic Origin				
		male	female	Caucasian	Black, not Hispanic	Asian/Pacific Islander	American Indian/Native Alaskan	Other

Subject Demographic Tracker
Name of Study

Total	Subject ID Num	Sex		Ethnic Origin				
		male	female	Caucasian	Black, not Hispanic	Asian/Pacific Islander	American Indian/Native Alaskan	Other
1	2-001	X			X			
2	2-002	X		X				
3	2-003		X		X			
4	2-004		X			X		
5	2-005	X		X				

Billing Tracker for Grant Charges

Name of study:
Subject ID number :

Visit	Test Name	Date of Service	Technical Fee	Professional Fee	Total	Notes
Screening						
Visit 1						
Visit 2						
Visit 3						
Visit 4						
Visit 5						
Visit 6						
Visit 7						

Name of study here

Subject ID number : 9-0004

Example of Billing Tracker for Grant Charges
imaginary costs assigned to example

Visit	Test Name	Date of Service	Techincal Fee	Professional Fee	Total	Notes
Screening						
	ECG	6-Feb-12	$ 300.00	$ 175.00	$ 475.00	
	specimen collection/ processing	6-Feb-12	$ 55.00	$ -	$ 55.00	
	pregnacy test	6-Feb-12	$ 100.00	-	$ 100.00	
Visit 1						
	pregancy test	7-Feb-12	$ 100.00		$ 100.00	
	Echocardiogram	7-Feb-12	$ 1,500.00	$ 1,800.00	$ 3,300.00	
	specimen collection/ processing fee	7-Feb-12	$ 55.00	$ -	$ 55.00	
Visit 2	NONE	14-Feb-12				
Visit 3						
	specimen collection/ processsing fee	21-Feb-12	$ 55.00	$ -	$ 55.00	
Visit 4		28-Feb-12				
	specimen collection/ processing	21-Feb-12	$ 55.00	$ -	$ 55.00	
Visit 5	NONE	6-Mar-12				
Visit 6	NONE	13-Mar-12				
Visit 7	NONE	20-Mar-12				
Visit 8	NONE	6-Apr-12				
Visit 9	NONE	6-May-12				

IRB #

Study name here

MASTER SUBJECT LOG

Subject Number	Subject Initials	Subject First Name	Subject Last Name	Contact Information	Phone Number	MRN	Date of Birth	Consent Type	Consent Version

IRB #
Study name here
MASTER SUBJECT LOG

Subject Number	Subject Initials	Subject First Name	Subject Last Name	Contact Information	Phone Number	MRN	Date of Birth	Consent Type	Consent Version
20-001	ALF	Albert L.	Friend	911 Pickled Pepper Drive Omaha, NE 68198	(xxx) 000-0000	Z9999	01JAN1900	Adult	v. 1.0 18MAY12
20-002	MAC	Mary A.	Card	346 White Fleece Road Omaha, NE 68198	(xxx) 111-1111	Z99899	02JAN1901	Proxy	v. 1.0 18MAY12

Study Name: **Screen Visit**

                                                        Subject Initials: _____ Subject ID Num - _____

                                            Room #

DATE (__-__-___): _____

Informed Consent Process	
The process of informed consent was conducted at _____ on _____ prior to the start of any study related procedures	Individuals present:
Questions asked by the patient and answered by the research personnel:	
Consent type	☐ adult ☐ proxy:
Copy of signed consent form given to subject	☐ yes ☐ no Reason:
Copy of Rights of Research Subjects given to subject	☐ yes ☐ no Reason:
Copy of consent placed in medical record	☐ yes ☐ no Reason:
Progress note in chart	☐ yes ☐ no Reason:
Consent version used:	

Research Coordinator: _____ Date: _____

Informed Consent Documentation Tool

Date: 13 AUG 11

The process of informed consent was conducted at ___2 pm___ on ___13 AUG 11___ prior to the start of any study related procedures	Individuals present: *patient, patient's spouse Mary Jones, Dr. Mark Rupp, Jen Cavalieri*
Questions asked by the patient and answered by the research personnel:	*Where are the study visits conducted? When will we know which drug dose we got?*
Consent type	(adult) proxy:
Copy of form given to subject	(yes) no Reason:
Copy of Education on Subject's Rights given to subject	(yes) no Reason:
Copy of consent placed in medical record	(yes) no Reason:
Progress note in chart	(yes) no Reason:
Consent version used: *Adult v1.0 16 MAY11*	

Research Coordinator: ___*Signature*_____ Date: ___*13 Aug 11*___

IRB #
SAE Summary Form

Study Name:

Subject	Event	Date of Event		Related/ Possibly Related/ Not related	IRB		Sponsor	Comments
		start	end	*per PI*	notified	response	notified	

IRB #528-10-FB
SAE Summary Form-example   Study Name here

Subject	Event	Date of Event		Related/ Possibly Related/ Not related per PI	IRB notified	IRB response	Sponsor notified	Comments
		start	end					
AAA-001	Bilateral PE	9-Jan-12	31-Jan-12	possibly related	9-Jan-12	6-Feb-12	9-Jan-12	
	worsening pancreatic cancer	31-Jan-12		possibly related	31-Jan-12	6-Feb-12	31-Jan-12	death
BBB-003	Hospitalization: intractable back pain	23-Feb-12	27-Feb-12	not related	23-Feb-12	8-Mar-12	23-Feb-12	
CCC-007	Bilateral DVT	25-May-12	31-May-12	possibly related	25-May-12	31-May-12	25-May-12	

This page intentionally blank.

Site Evaluation Visit

Name of study here	
Date of meeting here	

Purpose: Site evaluation visit

Requested items:

- Time for research questions with the lead clinical research coordinator (CRC)
- Tour of facilities
- Meeting time with investigational pharmacist: 30 minutes
- Meeting time with principal investigator: 30 minutes

Schedule:

0800–0900	Arrival, CRC will meet at xxx entrance, review of protocol logistics
0900–1000	Tour of facility (Clinic, radiology, laboratory)
1000–1100	Discussion of site logistics with research coordinator
1100-1130	Meeting with Investigational Pharmacist (protocol review, storage temp logs, etc.)
1130–1300	Continued discussion, working lunch with research coordinator
1300–1330	Meeting with principal investigator, review of protocol and investigator responsibilities
1330	Monitor to leave for airport

This page intentionally blank.

Study Reminder Checklist

Frequency	Task	Activity/document type
Daily		
	Check messages	Phone and email
	Temperature monitoring and documentation for research specimen or supply refrigerators or freezers	• Maintain temperature log on front of equipment. • File log in the regulatory binder.
	Carry out screening and recruitment activities.	• Use the study-specific inclusion/ exclusion criteria as a worksheet. • Communicate with referral sources.
	Conduct a high-level review of each clinical trial or project.	• What is happening? • What needs to be done? • What are we waiting to hear about or finalize?
Weekly		
	Check subject-visit log for each study for upcoming study visits.	• Verify accuracy of dates. • Update all current and estimated future dates.
	Conduct subject study visits.	• Complete source document checklists.
	Perform data entry.	• Check electronic database for queries and resolve. • Enter new data.
	Check supplies.	• Blood-collection kits • Office supplies
	Attend investigator update meeting.	• Update agenda with discussion items. • Update spreadsheet of current studies.
	Prepare for next week's meetings.	• Set up file folder. • Insert relevant documents. • Review attendee list. • Create agenda, including relevant items for discussion or decisions. • Send agenda to meeting leader or attendees as appropriate.
	Review and clear out email messages.	• Download electronic correspondence and place into intermediate filing.
	Do final filing.	• Choose one trial or project to do complete filing on.
	Check milestones.	• Check clinical-trial recruitment status: goals, screened, enrolled. • Check on upcoming deadlines for PI projects.
Monthly		
	Scheduled reports	• Complete reports.
	Check schedule for quarterly milestones	• Recruitment status on each clinical trial • Regulatory milestones • PI project deadlines
Quarterly		
	Reports	• Expect routine monitoring visits. • Update quality-control documents for each study. • Get recruitment status on each clinical trial. • Check regulatory milestones. • Verify PI project deadlines.

This page intentionally blank.

Weekly Report

	Status	**Notes**
Study A	Open, 3 active subjects/3 completed subjects	• Data Safety Monitoring Board meeting Friday • Potential subject in screening
Study B	Pending, regulatory, and contract approval in progress	• Working on source documents • Micro lab meeting Tuesday
Study C	Open, 12 active, 24 completed, 2 screen failures	• Monitoring visit Wednesday and Thursday • Protocol amendment coming • Monthly coordinator conference call Monday
Project #1	Week 4 of 6, total hubs sampled = 340	• Repeat lab cultures • Draft abstract for deadline 01 OCT 12
Time	Holiday 24 NOV 12	• CRC out 24–25 NOV 12 • PI on call and will cover active subjects

IRB# Name of Study: **Screening Visit Checklist**

Site # Investigator: **Subject ID Num** _____

Screening Visit Checklist
Date   **Time**
Vital Signs BP _____ Temperature _____ ☐ C ☐ F Pulse _____ Respirations _____
Medical History ☐ yes   **Concomitant Medication History** ☐ yes **Weight** _____
PI Physical Examination ☐ yes date _____ ☐ print dictated report
Allergies _____ ECG ☐ yes date _____ (w/in 28 days prior to randomization)
Laboratory
Serum pregnancy Test ☐ yes Result: _____ ☐ no reason: _____
Blood (Central Lab) Collection date ____ time _____ centrifuge time _____ shipped ☐ yes ☐ no _____
ECHOCARDIOGRAM
Scheduled Date   Time
Clinical procedure per hospital protocol. Data collection and de-identified CD of procedure:
Report of Results: _____ PI Review _____
Study Diary
☐ Education _____
Study Drug
☐ Education _____

Screening Visit Checklist

Date: _____ Time: _____

VITAL SIGNS BP _____ Temperature _____ C / F Pulse _____ Respirations _____

MEDICAL HISTORY yes   **CONCOMITANT MEDICATION HISTORY** yes   Weight _____

PI PHYSICAL EXAMINATION yes   date _____   print dictated report

ALLERGIES _____   **ECG** yes date _____ (w/in 28 days prior to randomization)

LABORATORY

Serum Pregnancy Test yes Result: _____   no reason: _____

Blood (Central Lab) Collection date _____ time _____ centrifuge time _____ shipped yes no _____

ECHOCARDIOGRAM

Scheduled Date _____   Time _____

Clinical procedure per hospital protocol.   Data collection and de-identified CD of procedure:

Report of Results: _____   PI Review _____

STUDY DIARY

Education _____

STUDY DRUG

Education _____

SPECIMEN

Collection supplies: Kit   Cool pac (store in freezer)   Instruction sheet   labels

DAY 1 APPOINTMENT

Date _____   time _____   clinic room scheduled

Urine collection cup for pregnancy test Visit 1 DAY 1   Collection supplies   Instructions

Randomization of Study Drug by Investigational Pharmacist   **Scheduled Pick Up** _____   Date _____   Time _____

Medical orders (specimen collection, pregnancy test) into medical record

TRACKERS

Subject Visit Log   Master Subject Log

Coordinator: _____   Date _____

Source Document Binder Contents *(customize this with study-specific information)*

Section	Description	Comments and tips
Front	Study Schedule of Events (SOE) (Shown in Chapters 3 and 6)	Readily available for reference. Recommendation: If the sponsor has not created one, or if this is an investigator-initiated trial, it is well worth the time for site personnel to create this.
	Demographic information	Print the medical record fact sheet listing name, contact information, next of kin, etc. OR Create a form and fill in this information
	Original signed informed-consent form and documentation of the process (Shown in Chapters 5 and 7)	This all-important document can be maintained in the subject's source documentation or filed in the study regulatory binder
	List of target study visit dates and/or calendar	Study-visit calendars are easy to create by going online and downloading a free blank template. Generally a monthly view works well. Placing 3 months on a page provides a valuable at-a-glance view of upcoming target visit dates.
	Site Visit Log (Shown in Chapters 4 and 6)	This log is useful for review of enrollment status, upcoming visits, and compliance validation.
	Stipend payments (Shown in Chapter 3)	This log is useful for tracking the stipend payment process.
Screening section	Inclusion and exclusion worksheet	This may be provided by the sponsor or can be created by copying the protocol into a new document. This is very useful to make notes on as subject eligibility is confirmed, and it should be signed and dated by the investigator.
	Site-Specific Screening Checklist (Shown in Chapter 7)	Customized checklists help research personnel keep track of study-specific tasks.
	Medical and medication records that support subject eligibility and medical condition	Could include medical records, notes made by the investigator from the physical exam, or study staff interviews with subject.
	Investigational Drug Talking Points (Shown in Chapter 7)	Education worksheets listing talking points with subjects about completing the study diary, administration of the investigational product, or what to report to study personnel Research personnel can check off each item as it is addressed and make notes.
Randomization section	Copies of the documentation received (e-mail or fax) noting the subject and/or drug randomization	

Section	Description	Comments and tips
Section for each visit 1–5	Site-specific visit checklists	
	Physician documentation	Dictated summaries of subject status, physical examinations, and communication with the medical monitor and sponsor
	Copies of specimen requisitions, shipping airbills, and tracking confirmation	Specimen requisitions may have stickers on the form that are to be attached to the specimen containers and the site record form or spreadsheet.
	Laboratory reports (signed, dated and noted as clinically significant [CS] or not clinically significant [NCS] by investigator)	One option is to keep the laboratory reports with the study visit information. Another option is to create a study-specific tab where all laboratory results are filed.
Concomitant medications	A listing of all medications of interest for the study. The protocol often defines the time period of interest, such as the previous 12 months, previous 7 days, etc.	This documentation could include medication references in admission or discharge summaries, medication administration records (MARs) from the patient's medical record, or a spreadsheet created by the sponsor or site personnel with such key information such as the name, dosage, frequency, and start and stop dates.
Echocardiogram	Sponsor instructions for specific data collection	
	Report results and any relevant medical orders	
Adverse event section	Subject tracker for AEs	Keeps track of adverse events of interest for the study. Allows for review of types, onset, and resolution of the events.
Serious adverse event section	Subject tracker for SAEs (Shown in Chapter 5)	Keeps track of report dates to the IRB and sponsor, onset, and resolution of the events.
	Each adverse event can be its own subsection and contain documentation from when the SAE was first discovered through IRB and sponsor notification, request for information from the sponsor's safety professionals, query resolution and additional information, and completion of the site documentation.	Keeps detailed documentation of the related information.

250

IRB#	Study:	**Investigational Drug Talking Points**
Site:	Investigator:	**Subject ID Num** _____

Date
☐ The study drug is in capsule form..   1:2 chance of placebo (no active drug)
☐ The study drug needs to be started 1 day after the Screening Visit
☐ The first dose will be administered during your research visit appointment. You need to take the remaining three doses for the day at 12 noon, 6pm and 10pm. *Show the subject the written instructions on the study drug package.*
☐ Do not open or crush the capsules. Swallow the capsule whole using any beverage you wish. There are no study related food or beverage restrictions.
☐ It is very important that you keep the empty study drug bottle. Please bring this with you for your next study appointment.
☐ It is very important for you to note the time you take your study drug in the diary. Always bring your diary with you for your study appointments.
☐ If you forget to take you medicine at your regular time, skip that dose and take the next regularly scheduled dose.
☐ Your next appointment is scheduled for _____. You will receive the study drug for that day at that study visit.
Call your study nurse at   if you have any questions

Coordinator: _____   Date _____

This page intentionally blank.

Journal Article Summary Sheet (blank)

Title of Article	
Author	
Study goal(s)	
Figures and Tables	
Any evidence of bias or confounding variables?	
Statistics	
Conclusion	

Journal Article Summary Sheet (example questions)

Title of Article	Why is this article of interest to the reader? Why was this article selected?
Author	Who are they? Where are they from? Any obvious conflict of interest?
Study goal(s)	Is this article worth reading? Find the goals to determine whether the article is relevant to the reader
Figures and Tables	<ul><li>Go to these after you have clarified the study goals</li><li>Find the table that describes the study subjects. This will contain some demographic data, such as male-female, etc. Is there a clear balance of the baseline characteristics between groups?</li><li>How many subjects were involved in the study? (Subjects being a relative term-the subjects may be sampled objects, patient rooms being studied, etc). If there is a small number of subjects, randomization may not equally distribute the subjects. If it is a very large trial, randomization should result in an equal distribution of baseline variables (similar baseline demographics, underlying co-morbid conditions, etc.)</li><li>The figures/tables should also give you some sense of the "generalizability" of the article.</li></ul>
Any evidence of bias or confounding variables?	Bias is when an outcome is favored as a result of sampling or testing error. Confounding or extraneous variables may mislead an investigator into thinking that correlations exist. In research, it is challenging to remove extraneous variables.
Statistics	Efficacy = the difference in outcome between groups. Find the reported "confidence interval" which indicates the magnitude and precision of the study. How big are the groups? Data with 95% confidence intervals (CI) are usually reported. Some people feel 80% is sufficient. p-value is an indicator of how likely it is that your outcome is due to chance. p-values are arbitrary, but generally 0.05 is regarded as a cut-off point.<ul><li>$p <0.05$ means there is a statistically significant difference</li><li>$0.05 < p < 0.1$ is a borderline statistically significant difference (trend)</li><li>$p > 0.10$ means there was no statistically significant difference.</li></ul>
Conclusion	Do you agree with the author(s) concluding statements (based on the data and methods utilized?) Are there other relevant events affecting the outcome/conclusions?

Index

A

accepting risk, 31
ACRP (Association for Clinical Research Professionals), 183
administrative duties, 18–19
administrative/clerical workflow, 148–153
    correspondence, 155–156
    documentation, 153–154
    reports, 153–154
        financial, 154–155
        progress reports, 155
        weekly reports, 158–159
    study closeout, 159–160
    Study Reminder Checklist, 152–153
    team communication, 156–158
administrator financial responsibilities, 38–39
adverse events documentation, 115
    SAE Summary Form, 117
ALCOA (attributable, legible, contemporaneous, original, accurate), 165
analysis, 11
appliction to IRB, 108–112
assessment, 11
assignment, 11
audits, regulatory responsibilities, 90–91
avoiding risk, 31

B

bias, 11–12
Billing Tracker for Grant Changes, 111
binders
    Financial Document Binder, 41
    Regulatory Document Binder, 88–90
    Source Document Binder, 170–172
biostatisticians, 23
bottom-up budgets, 45
budget, 42–45
    bottom-up, 45
    Budget Workbook Summary, 45–50
    contract and, 67
    expenses
        chargemaster and, 54–55
        pass-through, 55–56
    research labor data capture, 51–54
    shortfalls, site logistics and, 62–66
    SOE (Schedule of Events), 42–43, 47–48
    top-down, 45

Budget Workbook Summary, 45–47, 48–50
    chargemaster, 48
    effort log, 50
    Investigational Pharmacy Services, 60–61
    reference documents, 48
    sample, 57–61
    SOE (Schedule of Events), 47–48
    Tests and Laboratory Tests, 59

C

case control studies, 8
case reports, 7
case studies, 7
CDA (confidential disclosure agreement), 66
certification, 183–184
CFR (Code of Federal Regulations), 82
chargemaster
    Budget Workbook Summary, 48
    expenses and, 54–55
CHG (chlorhexidine gluconate) study, 62–66
clinical caregivers, 23
clinical laboratory personnel, 23
clinical staff, strategies for teamwork, 13–14
Clinical Trial Summary, 14, 15, 157–158
clinical trials
    definition, 3
    nicknames, 5
clinical workflow
    CRFs, 147–148
    IM (investigator meetings), 129–133
    medication administration, 146
    patients, 136
    regulatory start-up, 133
    site evaluation visit, 126–129
    specimen collection, 142–145
    study startup, 126
    study visits, 136–142
        follow-up activities, 146–148
    subject recruitment, 133–135
cohort studies, 8–9

communications
    administrative workflow, 156–158
    document organization, 175–176
compliance, 24
    HIPPAA (Health Insurance Portability and Accountability), 24
conclusions, 11
conflict-of-interest documentation, IRB, 121
confounding, 11–12
confounding variables, 11
consent forms, 112–115
continuing education, 184–185
contract specialists, 67
    financial responsibilities and, 38
contracts
    CDA (confidential disclosure agreement), 66
    CRO (contract research organization), 67
    CTA (clinical trial agreement), 66
    exhibits, 67
    indemnification, 67
    intellectual property rights, 67
    master agreements, 67
    study budget, 67
    terms, 67–69
correspondence, 155–156
CRCs (clinical research coordinators), 124
credentialing, 95–96
CRF (case report form), 81, 147–148, 169
CROs (contract research organizations), 19, 67
    regulatory responsibilities, 79
cross-sectional studies, 8
CTA (clinical trial agreement), 66
CV (curriculum vitae), 21

D

data, 164
    ownership, 166
    retention, 166–167

data integrity, 165–166
DHHS (U.S. Dept. of Health and Human Services), 82
    HIPAA, 83
documentation, 153–154
    CRFs (Case Report Forms), 169
    NTF (note to file), 169
    Source Document Binder, 170–172
    source documents, 167–169
    tools, creating, 172–175
documents
    correspondence, 155–156
    CRF (case report form), 81
    DSMB reports, 81
    Financial Document Binder, 41
    IB (investigator brochure), 81
        adverse events, 115
        protocol deviations and violations, 117–118
    IM (investigator meetings), 132
    IRB (Institutional Review Board)
        application, 108–112
        consent forms, 112–115
        SAE (serious adverse events), 116
        start up process, 103–104
        waivers, 116–117
    organization
        communications, 175–176
        filing, 176–177
    regulatory, 87–90
        checklist, 106–107
    Regulatory Document Binder, 88–90
    research protocol, 80–81
    source data, 81
    Source Document Binder, 170–172
    source documents, 167–169
    team communication, 156–158
DSMB (Data Safety and Monitoring Committees or Boards), reports, 81

E

EC (ethics committee), 82
ecologic studies, 7
effort log (Budget Workbook Summary), 50
EMR (electronic medical record), 170
endpoints, 11
equipment management, 27–29
    SOP example, 29
ethics committee (EC), 82
ethics training, IRB, 121
exhibits in contracts, 67
expenses
    chargemaster and, 54–55
    pass-through, 55–56
    stipend payments, 56

F

fabrication, 91–92
falsification, 91–92
FDA (Food and Drug Administration), 82
    website, 5, 6
feasibility process, 39–42
federally funded trials, 12–13
filing, 176–177
finance administrators, 22
finances. *See also* funding sources
    administrative view, 24–25
    administrators, 38–39
    budgets, 42–45
    contract specialists, 38
    Financial Document Binder, 41
    investigator and, 38
    money loss, 73–75
    outcome assessment, 71–72
    payment reconciliation, 70–71
    PI (principal investigator) and, 38
    research coordinator, 39
    study feasibility and, 39–42
    study sponsor, 38

Financial Document Binder, 41
financial reports, 154–155
focus
    losing, reasons for, 73–75
    maintaining, 34
fraud, 91–92
funding sources, 12–13. *See also* finances
    federally funded trials, 12–13
    investigator-initiated trials, 12–13
FWA (federal-wide assurance), 84

G

GCP (Good Clinical Practice), websites and, 5
GLP (good laboratory practice), 85

H

HIPPAA (Health Insurance Portability and Accountability), 83
    compliance and, 24
holding area for files, 176–177
human subjects, 4
hypothesis, 10

I

IB (investigator brochure), 81
ICH (International Committee on Harmonisation)
    regulations and, 82
    SOPs and, 25
    website, 5
IM (investigator meetings), 129–133
informed consent, 112–115
Informed Consent Documentation Tool, 114, 174
inspections, regulatory responsibilities, 90–91
intellectual property rights, 67
intermediate filing, 176–177
interventional studies, 3
Investigational Drug Talking Points, 172, 173

investigational pharmacists, 23
    roles, 125
Investigational Pharmacy Services (Budget Workbook Summary), 60–61
investigator, 22. *See also* PI (principal investigator)
    contract terms, 67–69
    financial responsibilities, 38
    IRB (Institutional Review Board), 100
    roles, 18, 124, 164
    secondary investigators, roles, 124
investigator-initiated trials, 12–13
IP (investigational pharmacist), regulatory responsibilities, 79
IRB (Institutional Review Board), 2–3, 99
    administrative personnel, 100
    conditional approval, 101
    conflict-of-interest documentation, 121
    continuing review, 105
    decline to review, 101
    documents
        adverse events, 115
        application, 108–112
        checklist, 106–107
        consent forms, 112–115
        protocol deviations and violations, 117–118
        SAE (serious adverse events), 116
        start up process, 103–104
        waivers, 116–117
    ethics training, 121
    fees, 121
    final approval, 101
    investigators, 100
    new study approvals, 101–108
    policies, 118–119
    relationship building, 119–120
    request for change, 104
    study closeout, 105
    tabled, 101
    withdrawals, 101

J–K

Journal Article Summary Sheet, 181
journal clubs for professional development, 180–182
Key Contacts List, 20

L

laboratories
    GLP (good laboratory practice), 85
    regulations, 85–86

M

masking, 11
master agreements (contracts), 67
Master Subject Log, 113
medication, administration, 146
misconduct, 91–92
mitigating risk, 31
monitors
    regulatory responsibilities, 79, 93–95
    roles, 164

N

networks, resources, creating, 72–73
new study approvals, IRB, 101–108
nicknames for studies, 5
non-human subjects, 137
NTF (note to file), 169

O

observational studies, 3
OHRP (Office for Human Research Protections), 84

P

participants, 4
participating personnel, 124
pass-through expenses, 55–56
payment reconciliation, 70–71
Payment-Reconciliation Log, 70–71
personnel, 19, 21–23
    files, 21
    Key Contacts List, 20
PHI (protected health information), 83
PI (principal investigator), 4. *See also* investigator
    financial responsibilities, 38
    regulatory responsibilities, 78
    roles, 18, 124
plagiarism, 91–92
policies, IRB, 118–119
population, 10
PPE (personal protective equipment), 137
professional associations, 183
professional development
    certification, 183–184
    continuing education, 184–185
    journal clubs, 180–182
    professional associations, 183
    research posters, 182–183
progress reports, 155
property management, 27–29
protocols, 4, 80–81
    deviations and violations, 117–118
    waivers, 116–117

Q–R

quasi-experimental studies, 9

RCTs (randomized, controlled trials), 9–10
reasearch team members, 4
recruiting subjects, 133–135
refrigerators, 28
regulations, resources, 5–6
Regulatory Document Binder, 88–90
regulatory oversight, 81–85
regulatory responsibilities
    audits, 90–91
    CFR (Code of Federal Regulations), 82
    credentialing, 95–96

CROs (contract research organizations), 79
DHHS (U.S. Dept. of Health and Human Services), 82
documents, organization, 87–90
FDA (U.S. Food and Drug Administration), 82
fraud and, 91–92
ICH (International Conference on Harmonisation), 82
inspections, 90–91
IP (investigational pharmacist), 79
laboratories, 85–86
misconduct and, 91–92
monitors, 79, 93–95
OHRP (Office for Human Research Protections), 84
PIs (principal investigators), 78
research assistants, 79
research coordinators, 79
research subjects, 78
roaming, 95–96
sponsor investigators, 79
sponsors, 79
regulatory specialists, roles, 164
regulatory start-up, 133
reports, 153–154
    CRF (case report form), 81
    DSMBs, 81
    financial, 154–155
    progress reports, 155
    weekly reports, 158–159
research assistants
    regulatory responsibilities, 79
    roles, 124, 164
research coordinator, 4, 22–23
    financial responsibilities, 39
    regulatory responsibilities, 79
    roles, 18, 124, 164
research labor data capture, 51–54
research posters for professional development, 182–183
research site, 4
research specialists, roles, 124
research subjects, regulatory responsibilities, 78
resources
    network, creating, 72–73
    regulatory, 5–6
resume. *See* CV (curriculum vitae)
retention of data, 166–167
risk management, 31–32
roaming, 95–96

S

SAE Summary Form, 117
sample documents
    Billing Tracker for Grant Changes, 111
    Budget Workbook Summary, 57–61
    Clinical Trial Summary, 157–158
    Informed Consent Documentation Tool, 114, 174
    Investigational Drug Talking Points, 172, 173
    Journal Article Summary Sheet, 181
    Master Subject Log, 113
    Payment-Reconciliation Log, 70–71
    SAE Summary Form, 117
    Schedule of Events, 154
    Screening Visit Checklist, 168, 172
    Site Evaluation Visit, 128
    Site Staff Task Delegation Log, 79–80, 165
    Site Visit Log, 95, 129
    Source Document Binder, 170–172
    Sponsor Payment-Remittance Detail, 70
    Study Reminder Checklist, 152–153
    Subject Demographic Tracker, 108
    Summary of a Clinical Trial, 72
    Weekly Report, 159
sample size, 10
Schedule of Events, 154
screening ratio, 135

Screening Visit Checklist, 168
secondary investigators, roles, 124
site contract personnel, 22
Site Evaluation Visit, 128
site evaluation visit, 126–129
Site Staff Task Delegation Log, 79–80, 165
Site Visit Log, 95, 129
SoCRA (Society of Clinical Research Professionals), 183
SOE (Schedule of Events), 42–43
    Budget Workbook Summary, 47–48
SOPs (standard operating procedures), 25
    document elements, 26
    research equipment example, 29
source data, documents, 81
source documents, 167–169
    NTF (note to file), 169
    Source Document Binder, 170–172
space. *See* workspace
specimen collection, 142–145
sponsor, roles, 125, 164
Sponsor Payment-Remittance Detail, 70
sponsors
    CROs (contract research organizations), 19
    financial responsibilities, 38
    regulatory responsibilities, 79
    roles, 18
    sponsor investigators, 79
    working with, 19
stakeholders, 19
stipend payments, 56
stress reduction, 34
study closeout, 159–160
study design
    analysis, 11
    assessment, 11
    assignment, 11
    bias, 11–12
    conclusion, 11
    confounding, 11–12
    confounding variables, 11
    endpoints, 11
    hypothesis, 10
    masking, 11
    sample size, 10
    study population, 10
study feasibility, 39–42
Study Reminder Checklist, 152–153
study types, 6
    case control, 8
    case reports, 7
    case studies, 7
    cohort, 8–9
    cross-sectional, 8
    ecologic, 7
    quasi-experimental, 9
    RCTs (randomized, controlled trials), 9–10
study visits, 136–137
    follow-up activities, 146–148
Subject Demographic Tracker, 108
subjects
    consent forms, 112–115
    informed consent, 112–115, 135
    non-human, 137
    recruiting, 133–135
    screen failure, 135
    screening ratio, 135
Summary of a Clinical Trial, 72
supplies, 30
supply shipments, temperature, 28

T

task delegation, Site Staff Task Delegation Log, 79–80
team members, 4
    communication, 156–158
    strategies for working together, 13–14
temperature, supply shipments, 28
Tests and Laboratory Tests (Budget Workbook Summary), 59

time-management, 32–33
tools, documentation, 172–175
top-down budgets, 45
transferring risk, 31
trusted websites, 5

W–Z

waivers, 116–117
websites
- FDA (Food and Drug Administration), 5, 6
- ICH (International Committee on Harmonisation), 5
- trusted, 5

weekly reports, 158–159
workflow
- administrative/clerical, 148–153
  - correspondence, 155–156
  - documentation, 153–154
  - reports, 153–155, 158–159
  - study closeout, 159–160
  - Study Reminder Checklist, 152–153
  - team communication, 156–158
- clinical workflow
  - CRFs, 147–148
  - IM (investigator meetings), 129–133
  - medication administration, 146
  - patients, 136
  - regulatory start-up, 133
  - site evaluation visit, 126–129
  - specimen collection, 142–145
  - study startup, 126
  - study visits, 136–142, 146–148
  - subject recruitment, 133–135

workspace, 30